Atlas of Neonatology

A COMPANION TO AVERY'S
DISEASES *of the* **NEWBORN**

Atlas of Neonatology

A COMPANION TO AVERY'S
DISEASES *of the* NEWBORN

DAVID A. CLARK, M.D.
Professor and Chairman
Director of the Children's Hospital at Albany Medical Center
Albany, New York

with contributions by

JEFFREY E. THOMPSON, M.D.
Executive Vice President of Gunderson Lutheran Medical Center
Director of Neonatal Intensive Care Unit
LaCrosse, Wisconsin

BRIAN M. BARKEMEYER, M.D.
Assistant Professor of Pediatrics, LSU Medical School
Director, Neonatal Intensive Care Unit, Children's Hospital
New Orleans, Louisiana

W. B. SAUNDERS COMPANY
A Division of Harcourt Brace and Company
Philadelphia London Toronto Montreal Sydney Tokyo

W.B. SAUNDERS COMPANY
A Division of Harcourt Brace & Company

The Curtis Center
Independence Square West
Philadelphia, Pennsylvania 19106

Library of Congress Cataloging-in-Publication Data

Clark, David A. (David Albert)

Atlas of neonatology: a companion to Diseases of the Newborn /
David A. Clark.—1st ed.

p.   cm.

ISBN 0-7216-7636-7

1. Neonatology Atlases.   2. Infants (Newborn)—Diseases Atlases.
   I. Avery's diseases of the newborn.   II. Title.
   [DNLM: 1. Infant, Newborn, Diseases—pathology Atlases.   WS 17 C592a 2000]

RJ251.C53   2000   618.92'01—dc21

DNLM/DLC   99–11887

ATLAS OF NEONATOLOGY   ISBN 0–7216–7636–7

Printed in the United States of America.

Last digit is the print number: 9   8   7   6   5   4   3   2   1

Preface

There is a disturbing trend in medicine to emphasize hi-tech diagnostic modalities without compiling a very thorough individual or family history or performing a proper physical examination. In the newborn, observation is critical, not only to detect subtleties that may lead to the diagnosis of a serious illness but also to counsel the patient's family on the many common, normal variations of physical findings. More than 25 years ago, it became apparent to me that the written descriptions of clinical findings in the existing textbooks of Neonatology were still inadequate to teach medical students, residents, and nurses. My budding passion for the photography of wildflowers was easily translated into a similar passion for photographically documenting the normal and abnormal physical findings of newborns. It was then a short step to supplement the story of an individual child with photographs of x-rays, ultrasounds, pathologic specimens, and intraoperative photographs. As in the collecting of stamps, the collection of clinical photographs is never complete, and a better-quality photograph to illustrate a particular condition is always being sought.

These photographs represent the experience and observations of but a few physicians. Many of the transient physical findings would never been documented without the helpful enthusiasm of nurses, house officers, and other professional colleagues. I, therefore, would like to thank all of the dedicated professionals who have been involved in the care of these children, many of whom were critically ill. Although the list is too numerous to mention individual names, without their encouragement, this atlas would not have been possible.

On a personal note, two physicians greatly influenced my choice to pursue an academic career and I would be remiss if I failed to acknowledge them. Dr. Floyd W. Denny, former chairman of the Department of Pediatrics at the University of North Carolina at Chapel Hill, was patient with a young pediatric house officer and provided a strong role model. Although his standards were high and his command of the information regarding the care of children was extraordinary, I most admired him for his ability to say "I don't know" and refer to another faculty member or community physician whom he thought would be more knowledgeable to answer that particular question. Once my decision to pursue an academic career was chosen, the possible paths were multiple. Dr. Ernest Kraybill, a new neonatologist, appeared on the scene in Chapel Hill and because of his gentle, kind, and compassionate role model as a neonatologist, within a few months my choice became obvious. I, with deep gratitude, wish to dedicate this book to these two excellent physicians.

DAVID A. CLARK

Contents

1 Maternal—Fetal/Neonatal

The successful development of a fetus is dependent not only on healthy genetic material, but also on the health and nutrition of the mother. Many recent advances in medicine have allowed women with chronic illnesses and severe metabolic disease (e.g., diabetes) to conceive and deliver neonates; many of these infants have unique problems relating to the illness of their mother. The use of fertility drugs has led to an increased incidence of in utero growth retardation and perinatal complications because of multiple gestation.

Fetal development obviously is not possible unless the placenta has become firmly established. Table 1-1 shows the time course of placentation.

The placenta has three crucial functions. It must first provide for transfer of essential nutrients from the mother to the fetus. Waste products such as urea, metabolic acids, carbon dioxide, and heat are transferred across the placenta and excreted by the mother. In addition, the placenta is a metabolically active tissue that synthesizes hormones important for the growth of the placenta and the fetus.

There are many causes of fetal growth retardation (Table 1-2) and growth excess. Although the large fetus is more prone to perinatal trauma, both large-for-gestational-age infants and growth-retarded infants more commonly suffer perinatal asphyxia and metabolic problems such as hypoglycemia.

TABLE 1-1

DEVELOPMENT OF THE PLACENTA

Day 6	Blastocyst attaches to endometrial epithelium
Day 7	Trophoblast differentiates into syncytiotrophoblast and cytotrophoblast
	Human chorionic gonadotropin
Day 8	Syncytioblast erodes endometrial tissue
	Blastocyst embeds in endometrium
Day 9	Blood-filled lacunae in syncytioblast
Day 10	Blastocyst sinks beneath endometrial endothelium
Days 11–12	Lacunar fusion
	Primitive uteroplacental circulation
Days 13–14	Primary chorionic villi
Day 21	Embryonic blood flowing in the capillaries of the chorionic villi
Weeks 4–18	Placenta thickens
Weeks 20+	Mature placenta covers 20%–30% of decidua

TABLE 1-2

CAUSES OF FETAL GROWTH RETARDATION

Poor maternal nutrition
  Low socioeconomic status
  Adolescent pregnancy
  Alcohol abuse

Poor fetal oxygenation
  Maternal hemoglobinopathy
  Maternal heart disease
  Tobacco use
  Altitude

Multiple gestation

Poor placentation
  Abnormal cord insertion

Maternal drugs and medications
  Phenytoin
  Warfarin
  Cocaine
  Narcotics

Transplacental infections

Chromosomal or genetic abnormalities

The length of the umbilical cord is determined by adequate amniotic fluid volume and fetal activity. Shortly after birth the cord begins to desiccate. If no antibacterial agent is used, the cord is shed at approximately 1 week of age owing to the activity of neutrophils drawn to the umbilicus by bacterial colonization. If the cord is not shed by 3 weeks of age, consideration should be given to persistence of a vascular supply, such as is demonstrated in many of the photos in this section.

Deficient amniotic fluid, either from poor production or prolonged leakage, may cause fetal compression features that commonly will resolve over time. However, decreased amniotic fluid with an associated increased amniotic fluid protein is a condition that predisposes to proteinaceous strands that transect the amniotic sac and lead to amputation of small parts.

The importance of prenatal life cannot be overestimated. Samuel Taylor Coleridge said it best when he wrote, "The history of man in the nine months preceding his birth will probably be far more interesting and attain events of greater moment than all the three score, ten years that follow it."

FETAL/PLACENTAL

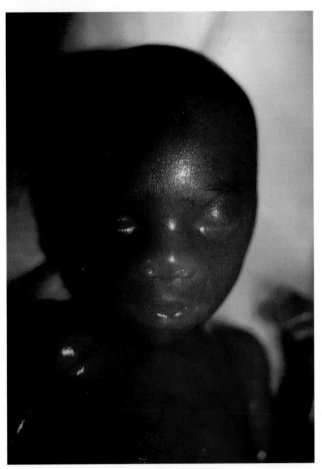

FIGURE 1–1. Fetus at 21 weeks' gestation

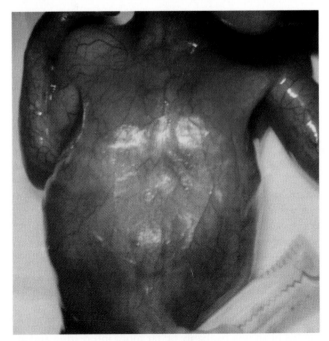

FIGURE 1–2. Fetus at 23 weeks' gestation

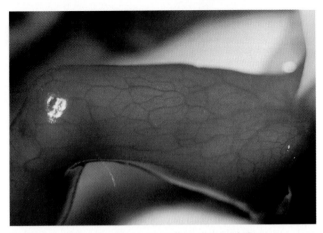

FIGURE 1–3. Vascular development. Leg of 23-week fetus

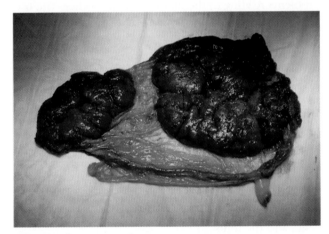

FIGURE 1–4. Accessory placenta

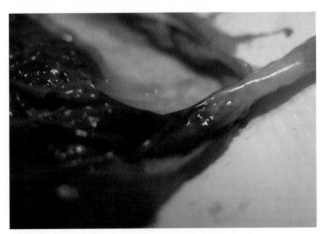

FIGURE 1–5. Marginal insertion of the umbilical cord

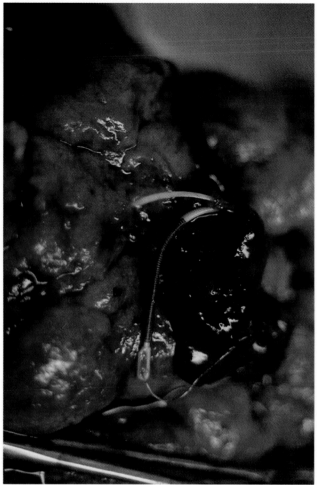

FIGURE 1–6. Placental abruption due to an intrauterine device

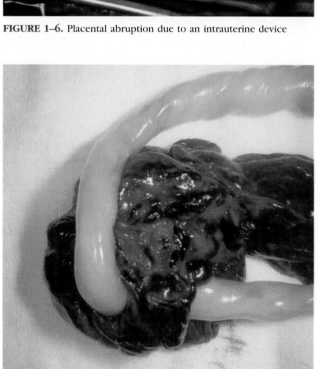

FIGURE 1–7. Placental abruption due to clot around the umbilical cord

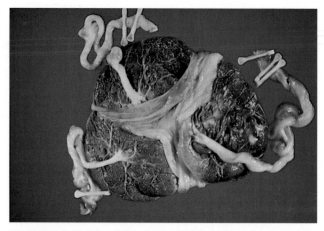

FIGURE 1–8. Healthy triplet placentas—fraternal

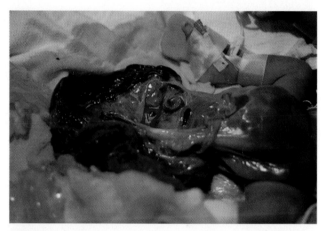

FIGURE 1–9. Abdominal wall defect with attachments to the placenta

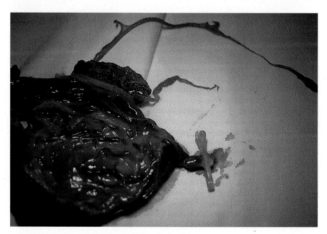

FIGURE 1–10. Aberrant umbilical artery-

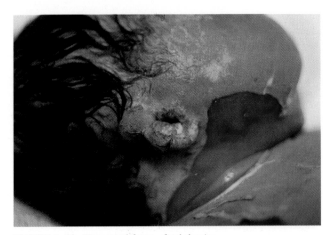

FIGURE 1–11. Macerated fetus—fetal demise

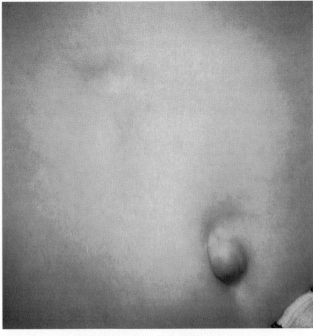

FIGURE 1–13. Abdominal wall healed at 10 weeks of age

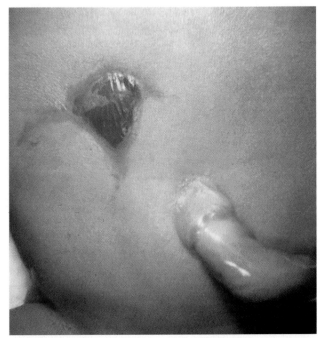

FIGURE 1–12. Abdominal wall necrosis due to extravasated blood from an intrauterine transfusion for Rh hemolytic disease

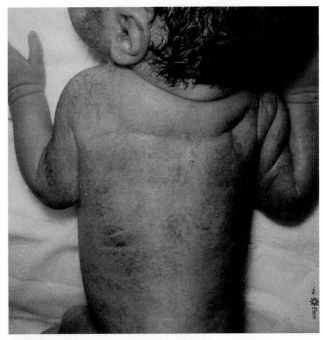

FIGURE 1–14. Blue vernix resulting from methylene blue injected into the amniotic fluid to detect a leak

PERINATAL TRAUMA

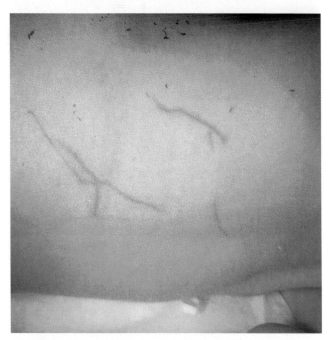

FIGURE 1–15. Back scratches from an amniocentesis

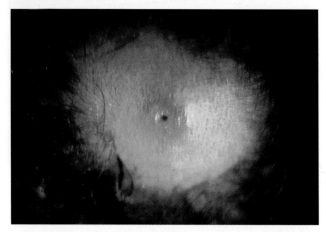

FIGURE 1–17. Scalp electrode trauma

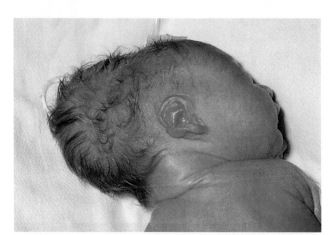

FIGURE 1–18. Caput succedaneum

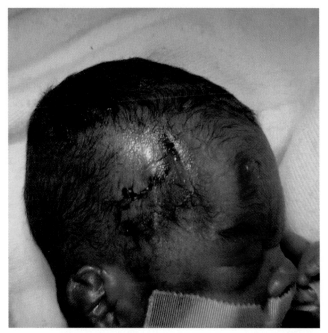

FIGURE 1–16. Scalp laceration from cesarean section incision

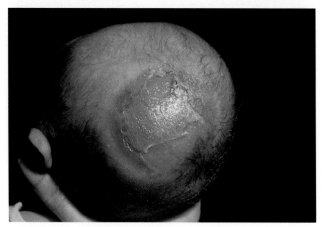

FIGURE 1–19. Scalp trauma from vacuum extraction

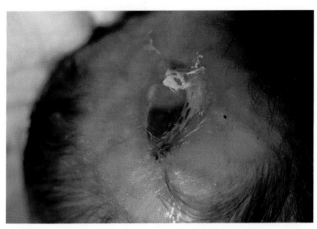

FIGURE 1–20. Scalp injury from an amniohook

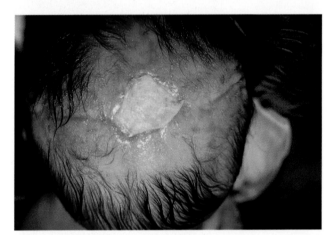

FIGURE 1–21. Allograft of scalp injury

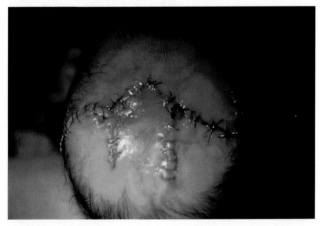

FIGURE 1–22. Surgical closure of scalp injury

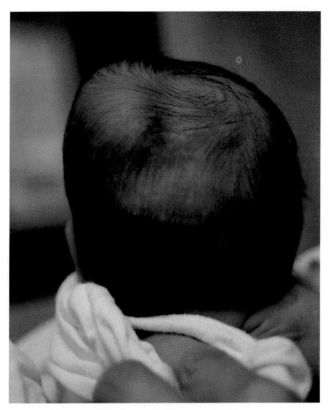

FIGURE 1–23. Left cephalohematoma

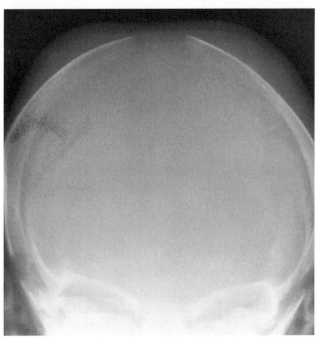

FIGURE 1–24. Skull radiograph of bilateral cephalohematoma

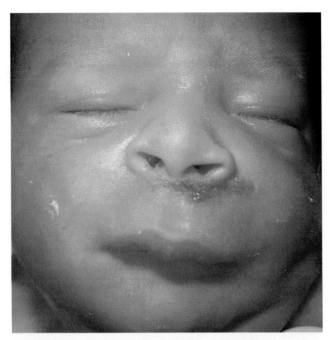

FIGURE 1–25. Facial trauma due to face presentation

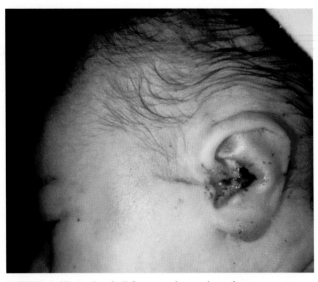

FIGURE 1–27. Basilar skull fracture—hemorrhage from ear

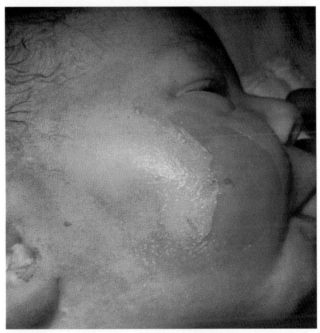

FIGURE 1–26. Facial abrasions from forceps

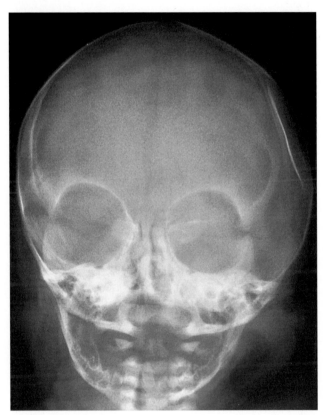

FIGURE 1–28. Skull fracture—radiograph

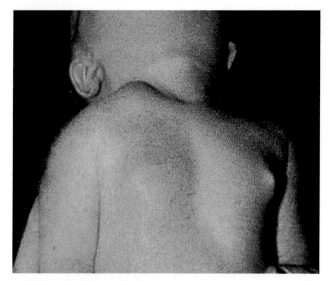

FIGURE 1–29. Fractured right clavicle

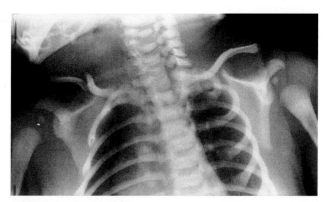

FIGURE 1–30. Radiograph of fractured right clavicle

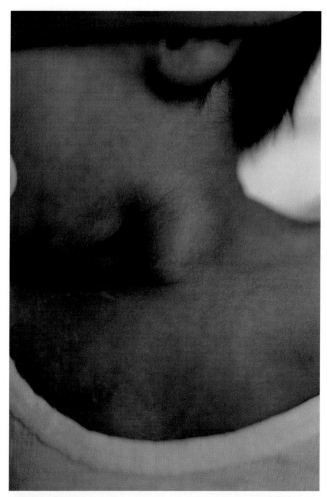

FIGURE 1–31. Hemorrhage into the sternocleidomastoid muscle

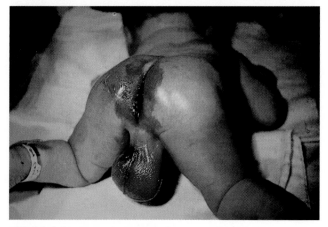

FIGURE 1–32. Perineal trauma, breech presentation

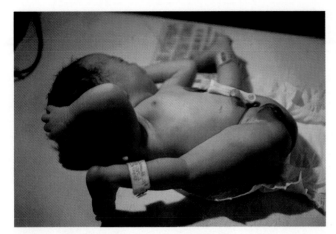

FIGURE 1–33. Breech presentation—hip laxity

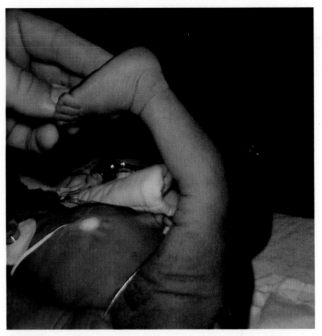

FIGURE 1–34. Genu recurvatum due to in utero positioning

GESTATIONAL AGE—PHYSICAL CHARACTERISTICS

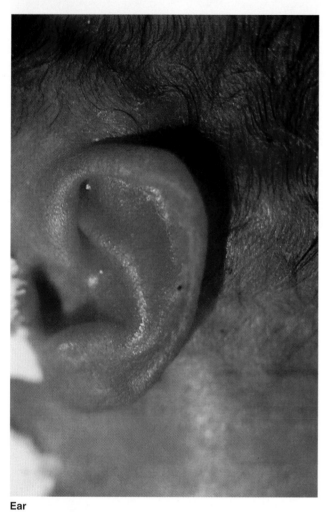

Ear

FIGURE 1–35. 28 weeks' gestation: little cartilage, pliable

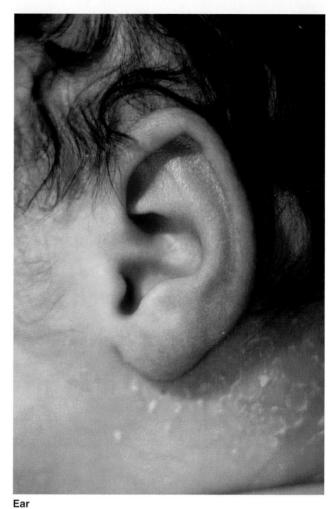

Ear

FIGURE 1–37. 36 weeks to term gestation: firm ear, well-formed margin

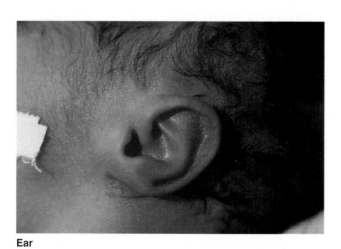

Ear

FIGURE 1–36. 32 weeks' gestation: increased cartilage, in-curving of outer pinna

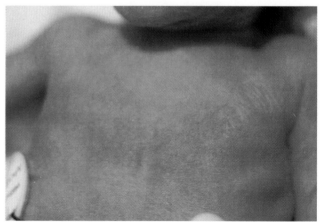

Breast

FIGURE 1–38. 28 weeks' gestation: no breast tissue, areola barely visible

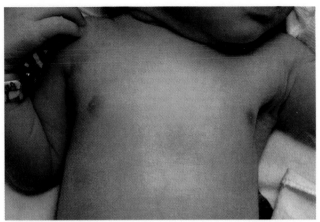

Breast

FIGURE 1–39. 32 weeks' gestation: visible areola, little breast tissue

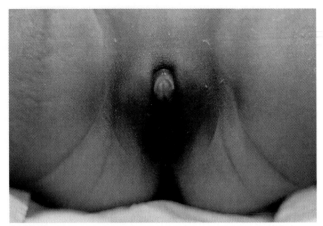

Genitalia

FIGURE 1–42. Female at 32 weeks' gestation: increased fat deposition in labia majora

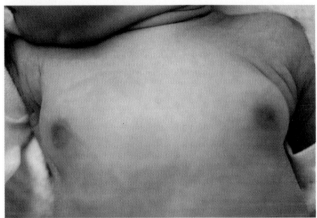

Breast

FIGURE 1–40. 36 weeks to term gestation: well-defined areola, breast nodules

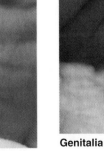

Genitalia

FIGURE 1–41. Female at 28 weeks' gestation: prominent clitoris, small labia majora

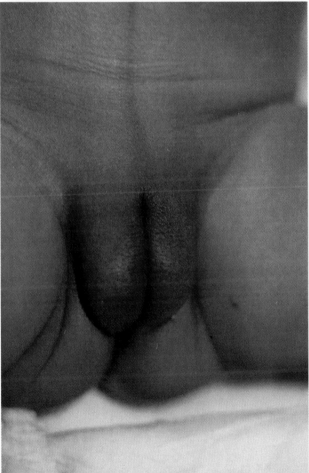

Genitalia

FIGURE 1–43. Female at 36 weeks to term gestation: labia majora nearly covering labia minora

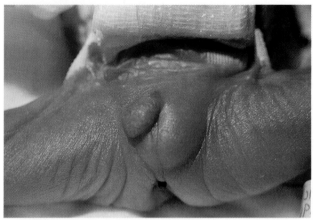

Genitalia

FIGURE 1–44. Male at 28 weeks' gestation: testes high in scrotum

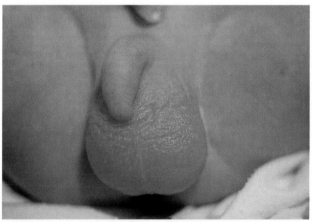

Genitalia

FIGURE 1–45. Male at 32 weeks' gestation: testes descending, some scrotal rugae

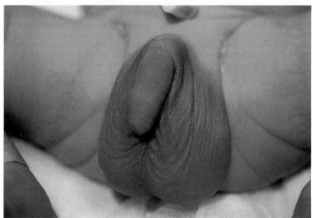

Genitalia

FIGURE 1–46. Male at 36 weeks to term gestation: testes well descended, increased scrotal pigmentation

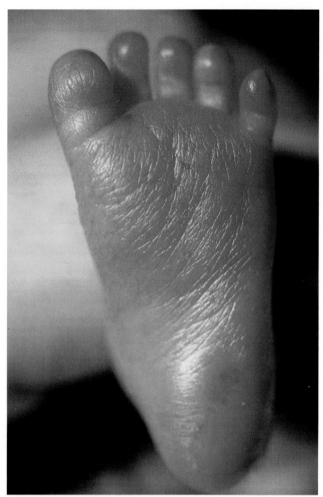

Foot Sole Creases

FIGURE 1–47. 28 weeks' gestation: smooth sole

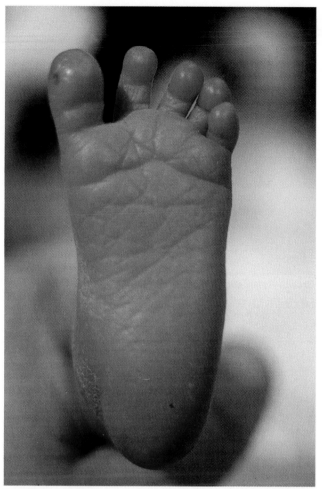

Foot Sole Creases

FIGURE 1–48. 32 weeks' gestation: creases in anterior one third

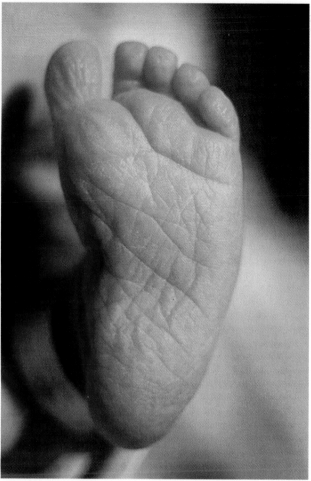

Foot Sole Creases

FIGURE 1–49. 36 weeks to term gestation: creases over the majority of the sole

GROWTH IN UTERO

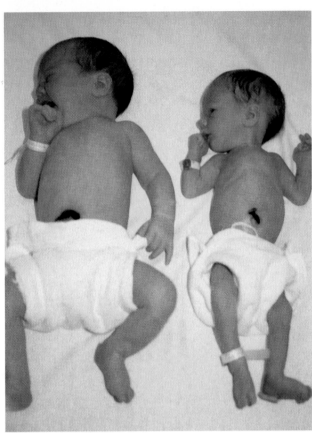

Growth Retardation

FIGURE 1–50. Discordant twins

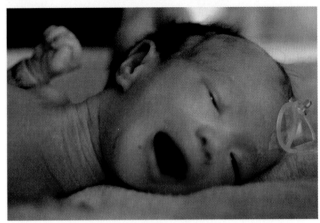

Growth Retardation

FIGURE 1–52. Small for gestational age: in utero infection

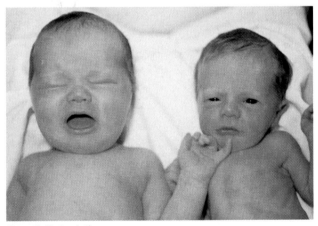

Growth Retardation

FIGURE 1–51. Discordant twins

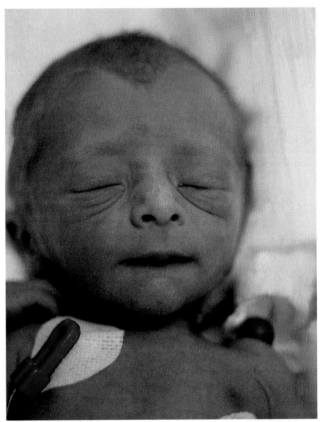

Growth Retardation

FIGURE 1–53. Small for gestational age: maternal hypertension

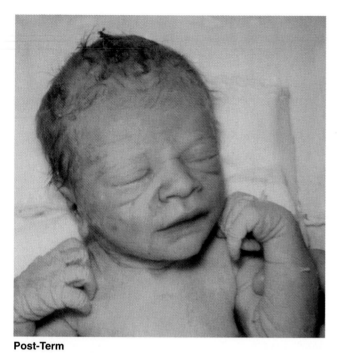

Post-Term

FIGURE 1–54. Wizened facies

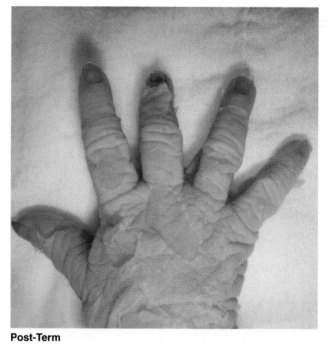

Post-Term

FIGURE 1–56. Long nails, peeling skin

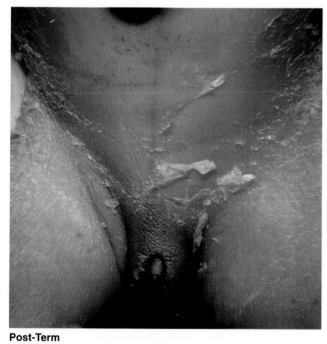

Post-Term

FIGURE 1–55. Peeling skin, loss of vernix

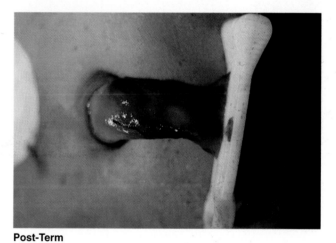

Post-Term

FIGURE 1–57. Meconium-stained cord

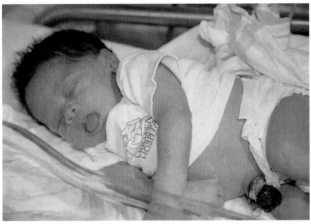

Growth Excess

FIGURE 1–58. Beckwith-Wiedemann syndrome: large for gestational age, protruding tongue, omphalocele

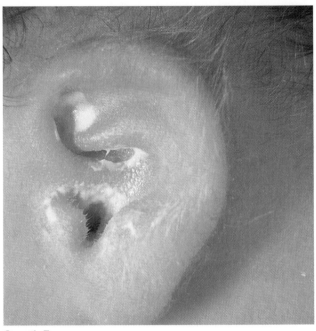

Growth Excess

FIGURE 1–60. Infant of diabetic mother: hairy ear

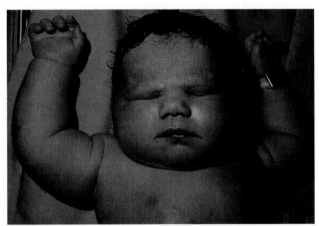

Growth Excess

FIGURE 1–59. Infant of diabetic mother: macrosomia

UMBILICAL CORD

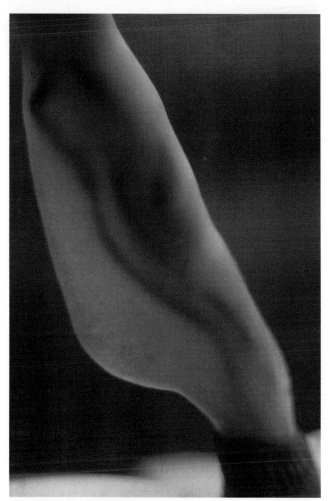

FIGURE 1–61. Transillumination: 3 umbilical vessels, 2 arteries, 1 vein

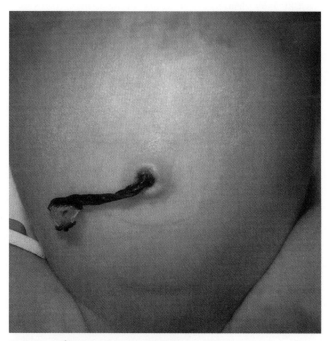

FIGURE 1–62. Normal drying umbilical cord

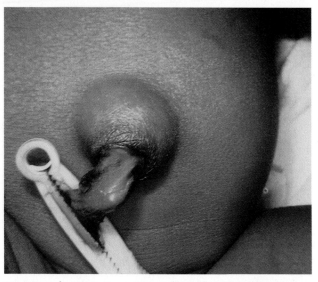

FIGURE 1–63. Triple dye staining of the cord; umbilical hernia

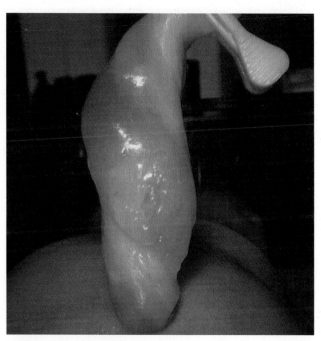

FIGURE 1–64. Excess Wharton's jelly

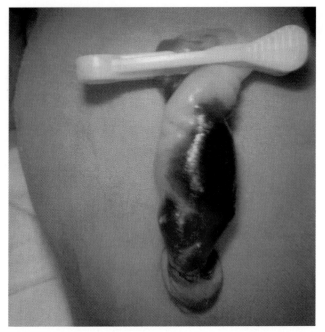

FIGURE 1–65. Cord hematoma

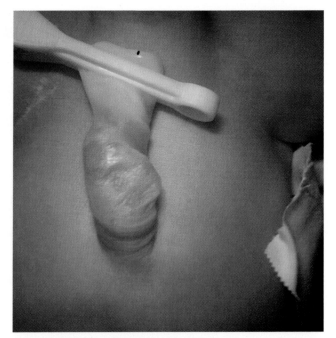

FIGURE 1–67. Excess skin

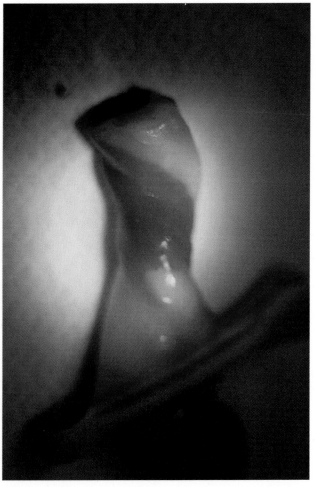

FIGURE 1–66. Cord vessel rupture

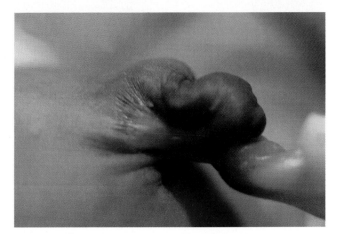

FIGURE 1–68. Hemangioma at the base of the cord

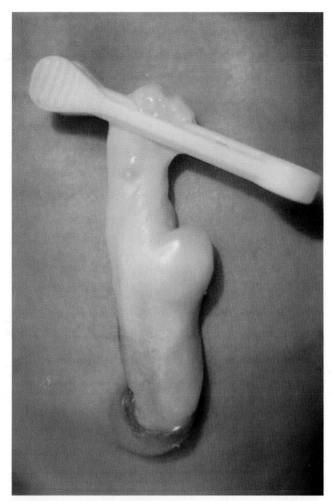

FIGURE 1–69. Cord hemangioma

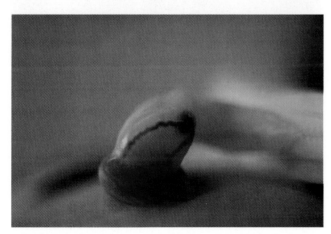

FIGURE 1–70. Arteriovenous malformation, cutaneous artery to umbilical vein

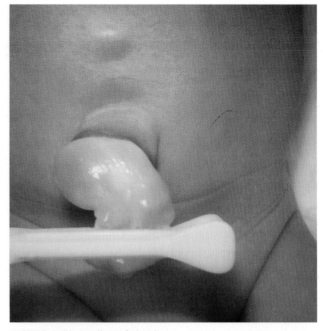

FIGURE 1–71. Small omphalocele-

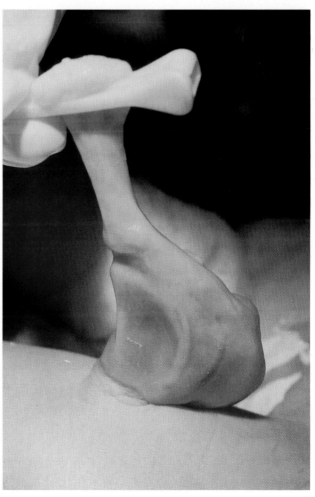

FIGURE 1–72. Sliding omphalocele

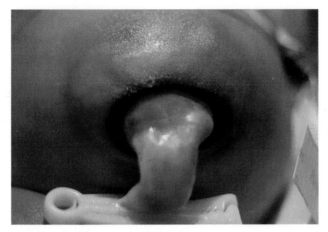

FIGURE 1–73. Massive umbilical hernia

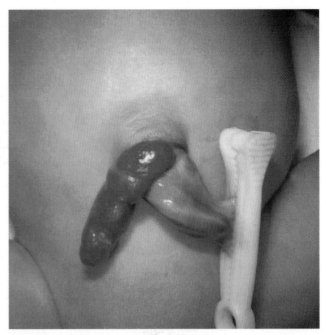

FIGURE 1–75. Ectopic colon

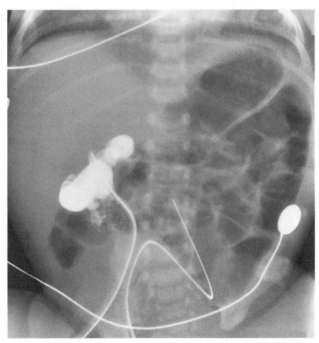

FIGURE 1–74. Radiograph of omphalomesenteric remnant filled with contrast

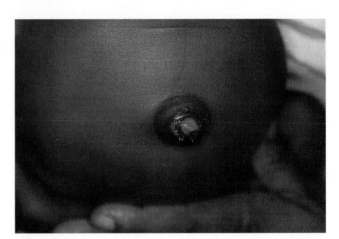

FIGURE 1–76. Umbilical granuloma

DEFORMATIONS DUE TO OLIGOHYDRAMNIOS

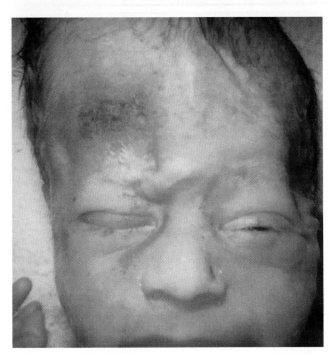

FIGURE 1–77. In utero head compression

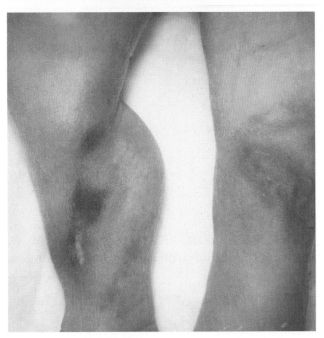

FIGURE 1–79. In utero compression of legs resulting in vascular compromise

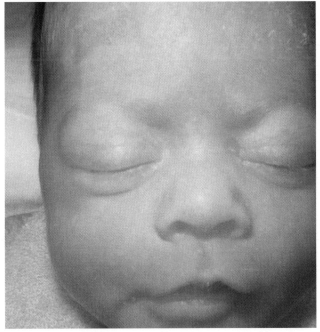

FIGURE 1–78. Healed head after 6 weeks

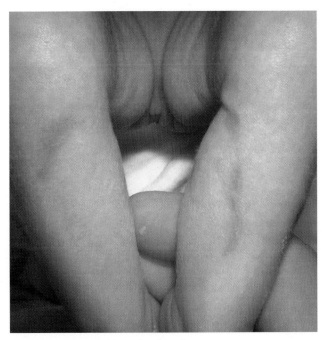

FIGURE 1–80. Healed legs after 6 weeks

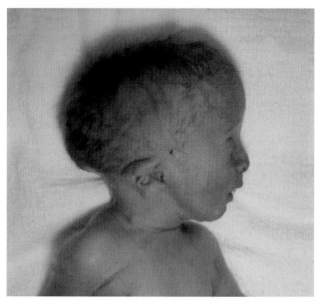

FIGURE 1–81. Facial compression: oligohydramnios due to renal agenesis

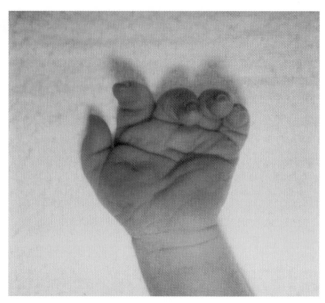

FIGURE 1–82. Broad, flattened hands

AMNIOTIC BANDS—DISRUPTIONS

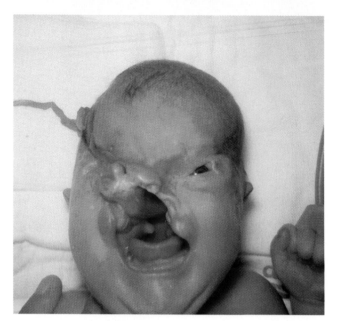

FIGURE 1–83. Facial disruption

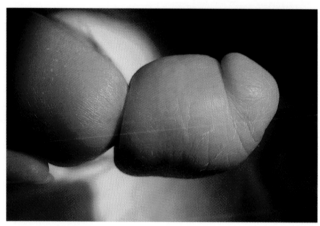

FIGURE 1–84. Hand: amputation

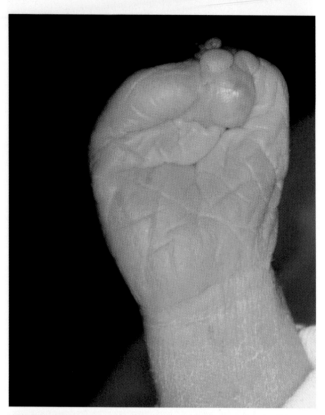

FIGURE 1–85. Hand: stubs of amputated fingers wrapped with an amniotic band

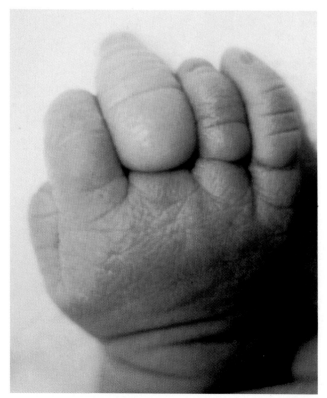

FIGURE 1–86. Hand: multiple amniotic bands

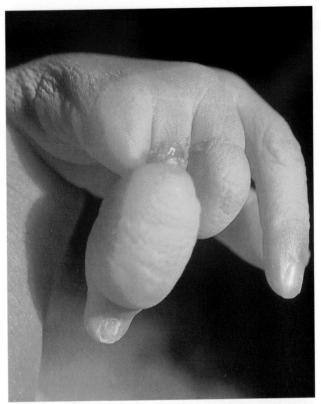

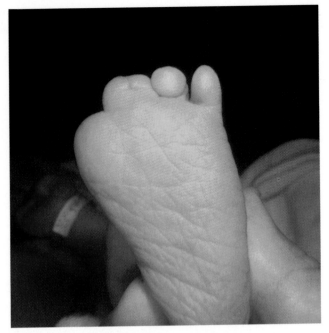

FIGURE 1–89. Amputated great toe

FIGURE 1–87. Hand: amputated fifth finger, edematous fourth finger with an amniotic band

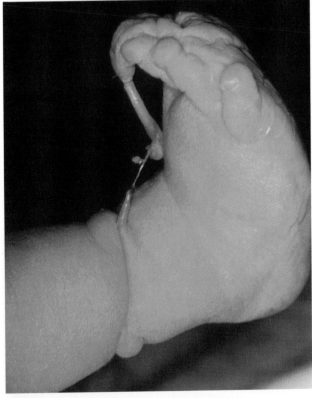

FIGURE 1–88. Foot with nail evulsion of great toe

CONJOINED TWINS

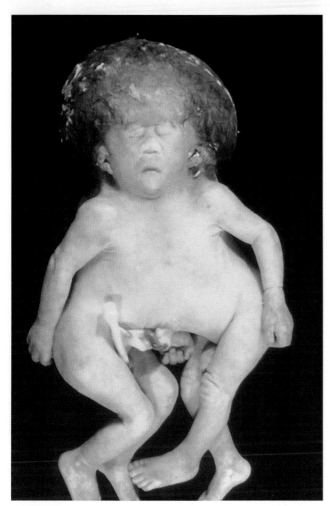

FIGURE 1–90. Janiceps, anterior view

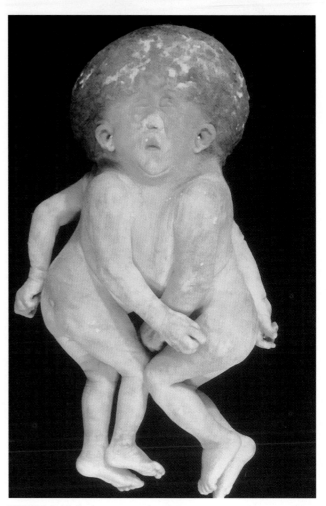

FIGURE 1–91. Janiceps, posterior view

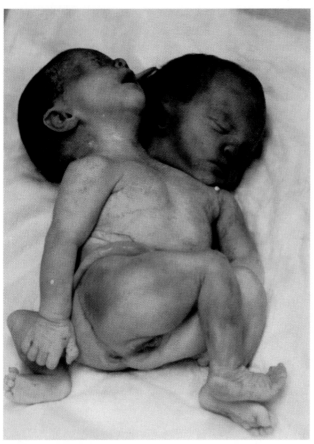

FIGURE 1–92. Double head

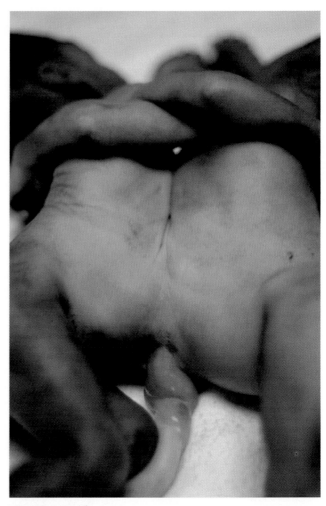

FIGURE 1–93. Thoracopagus

MATERNAL DRUGS—FETAL EFFECTS

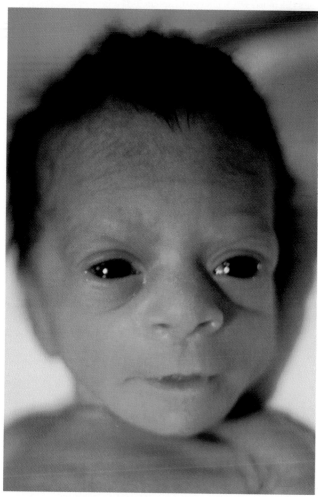

FIGURE 1–94. Fetal alcohol syndrome facies—long, flat philtrum, thin upper lip, short palpebral fissures

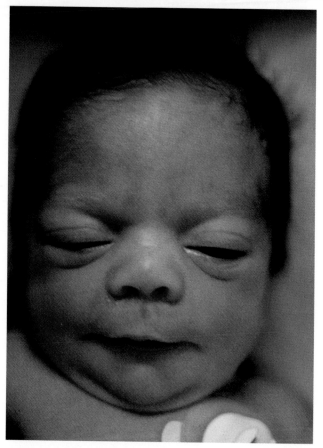

FIGURE 1–95. Fetal hydantoin syndrome facies

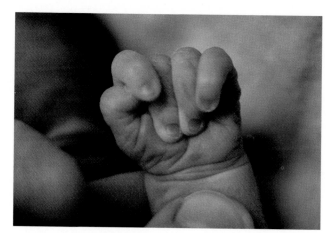

FIGURE 1–96. Fetal hydantoin syndrome—nail hypoplasia

SELECTED REFERENCES

Creasy RK and Resnik R. (1994) Maternal-Fetal Medicine, 3rd ed. Philadelphia, WB Saunders, Chapters 3-6.

Jones KL. (1997) Smith's Recognizable Patterns of Human Malformation, 5th ed. Philadelphia, WB Saunders.

Moore KL and Persaud TVN. (1998) The Developing Human: Clinically Oriented Embryology, 6th ed. Philadelphia, WB Saunders, Chapters 2, 3, 4, and 7.

Polin RA and Fox WW. (1998) Fetal and Neonatal Physiology, 2nd ed. Philadelphia, WB Saunders, Chapters 5-11.

Taeusch HW and Ballard RA. (1998) Avery's Diseases of the Newborn, 7th ed. Philadelphia, WB Saunders, Chapters 6-9.

2 Syndromes/Genetics

A congenital malformation is a significant defect in structure or function that exists in the fetus prior to birth. It may be from the time of conception or from an insult that occurs to the developing embryo or fetus during the course of gestation. This damage may persist and be irreversible. In general, the more genetic material affected, the greater the insult as more organ systems may be malformed. The chromosomal anomalies with multiple organ systems affected are those easiest to detect and are represented by photographs in this section. The incidence of common chromosomal abnormalities is enumerated in Table 2–1. Many chromosomal abnormalities, especially trisomy with the larger chromosomes and in-

TABLE 2–1

INCIDENCE OF COMMON CHROMOSOMAL ABNORMALITIES	
Trisomy 21 (Down syndrome)	1/660 newborns overall (incidence increases with maternal age)
Trisomy 18	3/1000 live births
Trisomy 13	1/5000 live births
XYY syndrome	1/840 males
XXY syndrome (Klinefelter syndrome)	1/500 males
XXX syndrome	1/1000 females
XO syndrome (Turner syndrome)	1/2000 females

TABLE 2–2

FREQUENCY OF GENETIC DISEASE AND MALFORMATIONS	
	%
Chromosomal disorders	0.5
Gene disorders	1
Congenital malformations	2–5
Minor anomalies	10–15

cluding triploidy, are aborted commonly in the first trimester.

Chromosome disorders account for only 0.5% of detected genetic disease (Table 2–2). Easily recognizable gene disorders account for approximately twice as many anomalies. Other significant congenital malformations have an incidence of approximately 2% to 5% and may be multifactorial, including a genetic component with an environmental factor. In addition, many other minor anomalies are not life-threatening or do not affect organ function and can be seen in as high as 15% of all neonates.

Maternal illnesses, such as diabetes, transplacental viral infection, in utero drug exposure, and maternal fever, have all been implicated in congenital malformations, especially if the problem is acutely suffered during the first trimester.

CHROMOSOMAL MALFORMATIONS

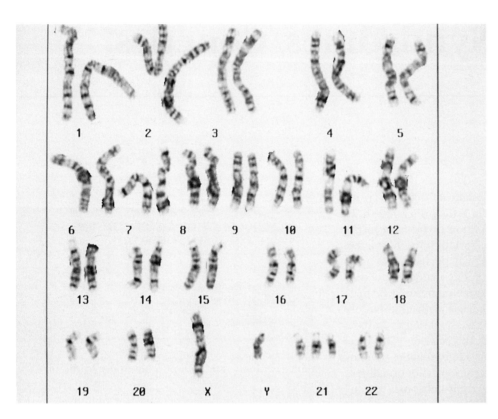

Trisomy 21 (Down Syndrome)

FIGURE 2–1. Karyotype:
47,XY,+21

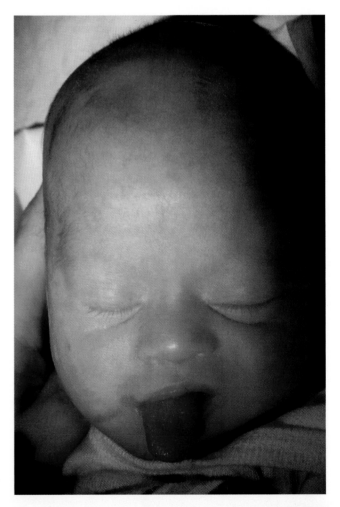

Trisomy 21 (Down Syndrome)

FIGURE 2–2. Face of a term infant with epicanthal folds and protruding tongue

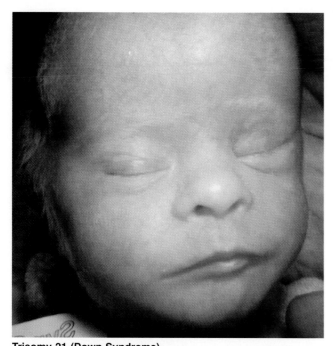

Trisomy 21 (Down Syndrome)

FIGURE 2–3. Face of a preterm infant, 32 weeks' gestation

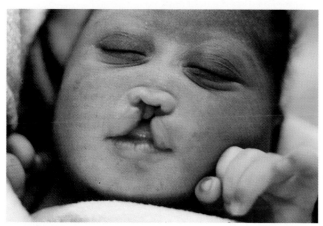

Trisomy 21 (Down Syndrome)

FIGURE 2–4. Cleft lip and palate

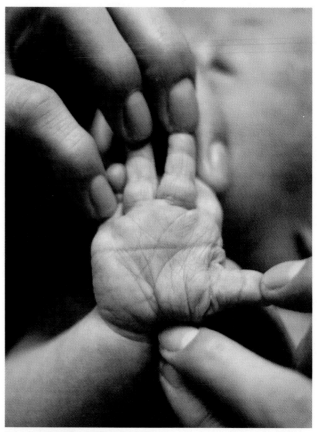

Trisomy 21 (Down Syndrome)

FIGURE 2–5. Simian crease

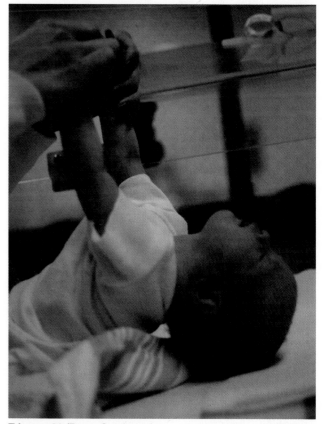

Trisomy 21 (Down Syndrome)

FIGURE 2–6. Hypotonia—severe head lag

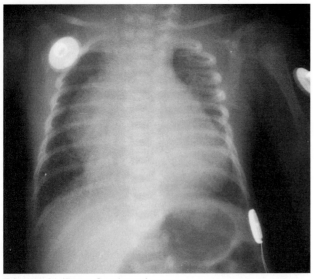

Trisomy 21 (Down Syndrome)

FIGURE 2–7. Chest radiograph—cardiomegaly due to an endocardial cushion defect

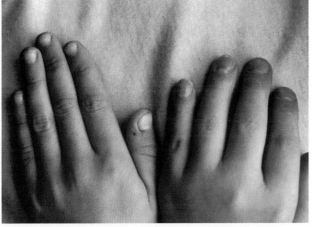

Trisomy 21 (Down Syndrome)

FIGURE 2–8. Clubbing of fingers in a 3 year old child with an endocardial cushion defect (right) compared with those of a healthy child (left)

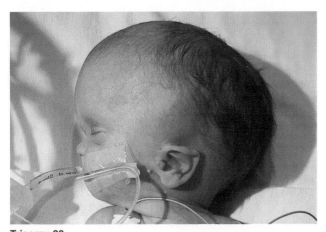

Trisomy 22

FIGURE 2–9. Macrocephaly

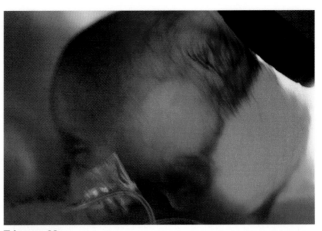

Trisomy 22

FIGURE 2–10. Transillumination of hydrocephalus

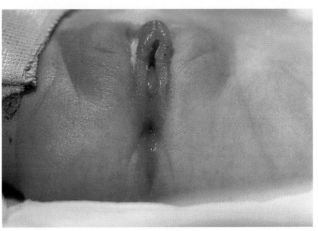

Trisomy 22

FIGURE 2–11. Anteriorly displaced anus

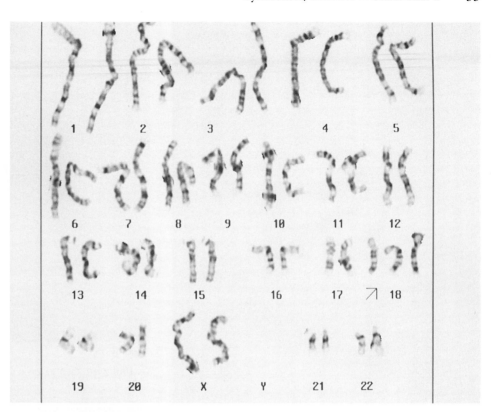

Trisomy 18

FIGURE 2–12. Karyotype: 47,XX,+18

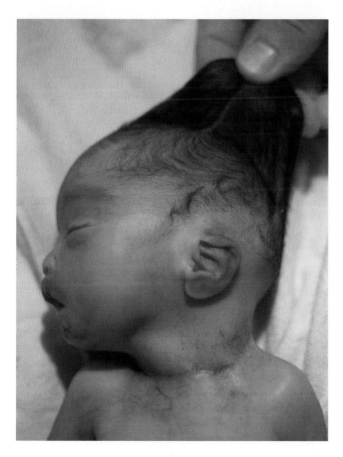

Trisomy 18

FIGURE 2–13. Redundant scalp

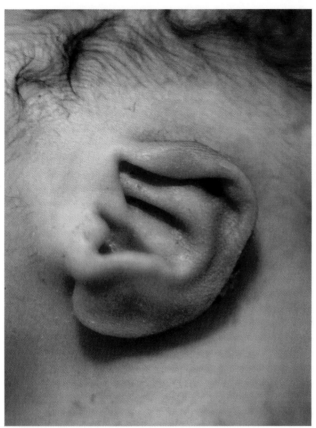

Trisomy 18

FIGURE 2–14. Malformed ear

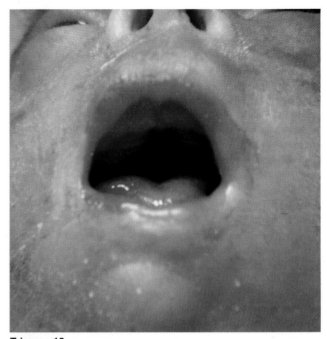

Trisomy 18

FIGURE 2–16. Cleft palate

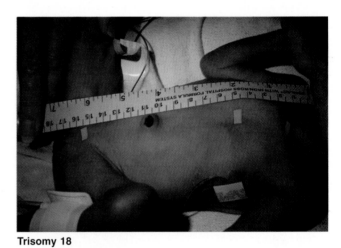

Trisomy 18

FIGURE 2–17. Short sternum

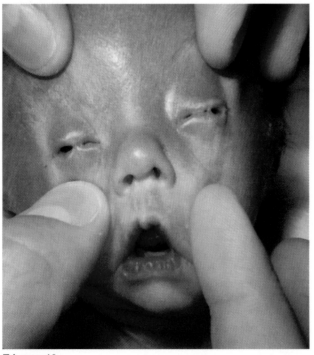

Trisomy 18

FIGURE 2–15. Partial fusion of eyelids

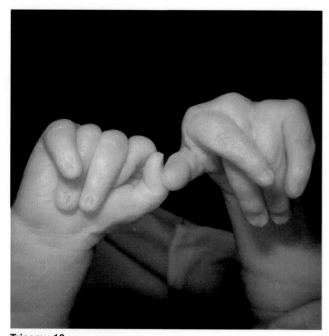

Trisomy 18

FIGURE 2–18. Clinodactyly

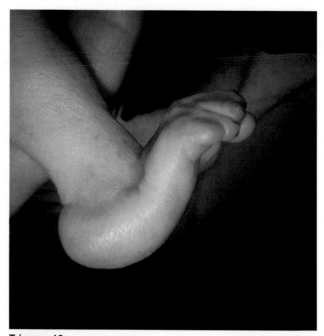

Trisomy 18

FIGURE 2–20. Rocker-bottom foot

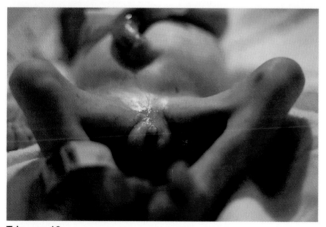

Trisomy 18

FIGURE 2–19. Limited hip abduction

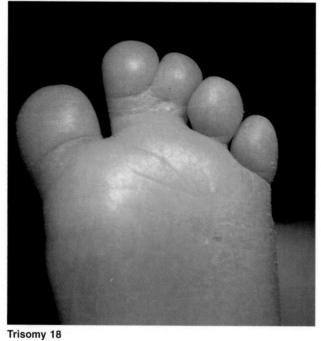

Trisomy 18

FIGURE 2–21. Syndactyly

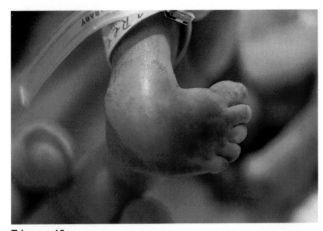

Trisomy 18

FIGURE 2–22. Severe equinovarus

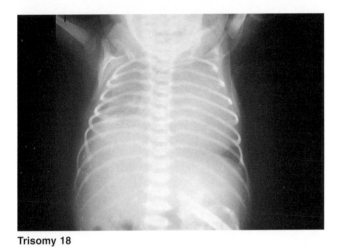

Trisomy 18

FIGURE 2–23. Chest radiograph: incomplete ossification of right clavicle, cardiomegaly

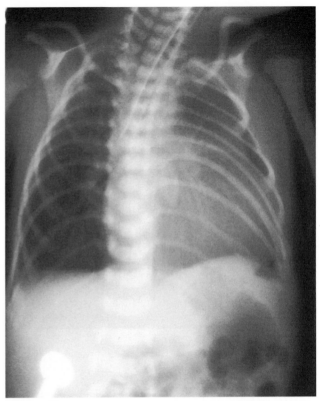

Trisomy 18

FIGURE 2–24. Chest radiograph: complex congenital heart disease, thin ribs

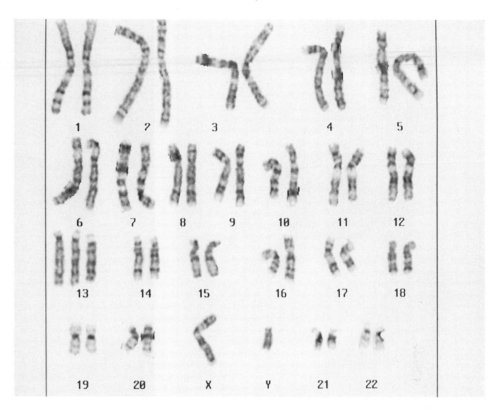

Trisomy 13

FIGURE 2–25. Karyotype: 47,XY,+13

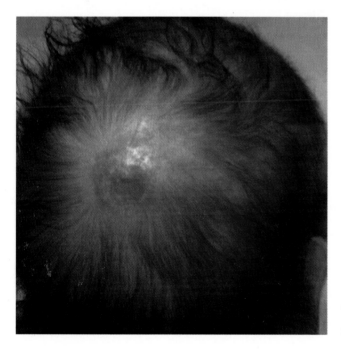

Trisomy 13

FIGURE 2–26. Scalp defect

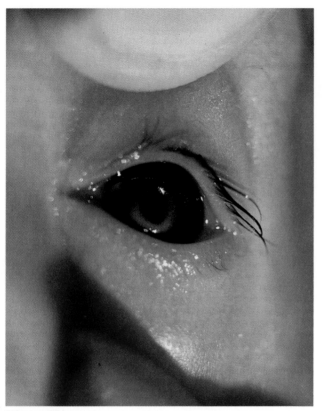

Trisomy 13

FIGURE 2–27. Abnormal cornea

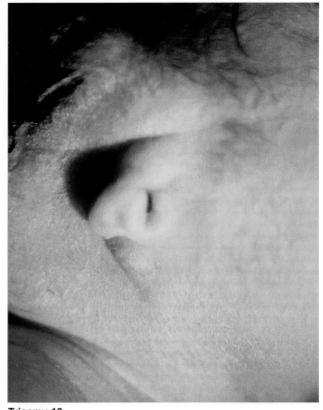

Trisomy 13

FIGURE 2–29. Folded, hypoplastic pinna

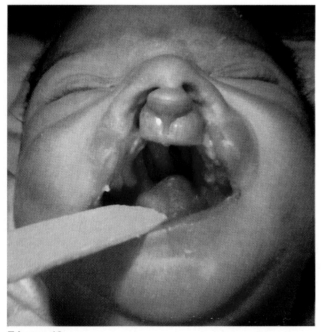

Trisomy 13

FIGURE 2–28. Cleft lip/palate

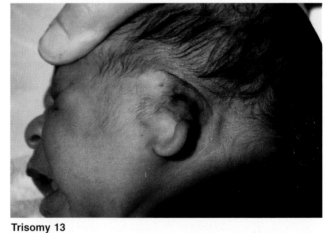

Trisomy 13

FIGURE 2–30. Aplastic pinna

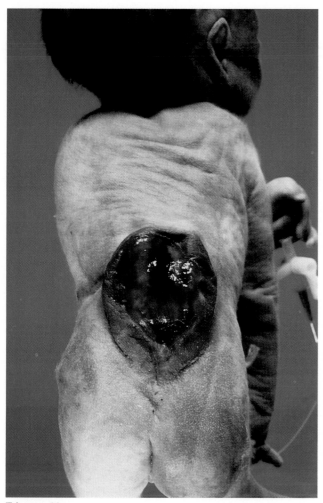

Trisomy 13

FIGURE 2–31. Meningomyelocele

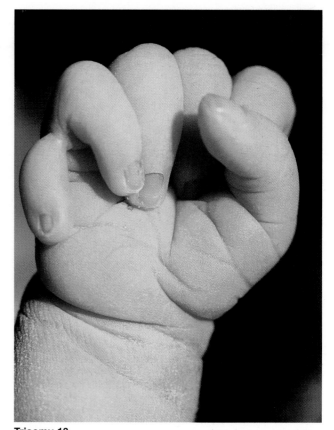

Trisomy 13

FIGURE 2–32. Postaxial polydactyly

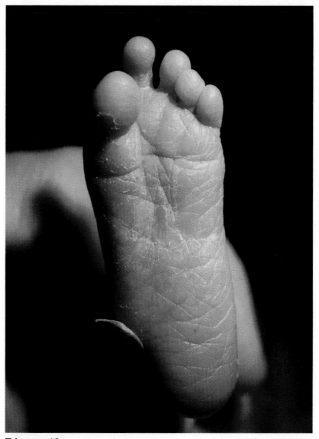

Trisomy 13

FIGURE 2–33. Midfoot hypoplasia

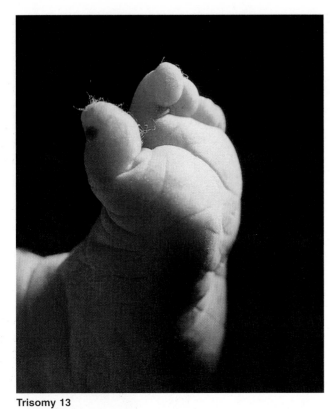

Trisomy 13

FIGURE 2–34. Cocked-back great toe, cleft between hallus and second toe

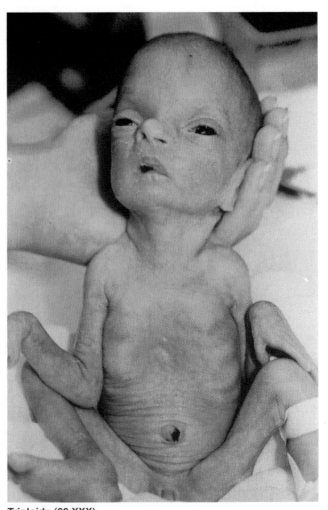

Triploidy (69,XXX)

FIGURE 2–35. Severe growth retardation, hypertelorism

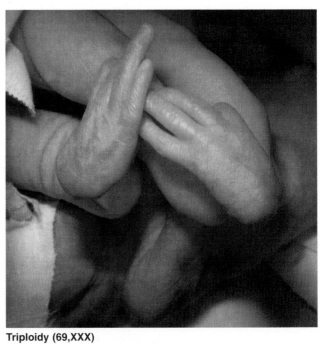

Triploidy (69,XXX)

FIGURE 2–36. Hypoplastic hands with flexion contractures

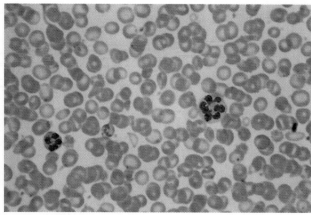

Triploidy (69,XXX)

FIGURE 2–38. Peripheral smear—neutrophil hypersegmentation

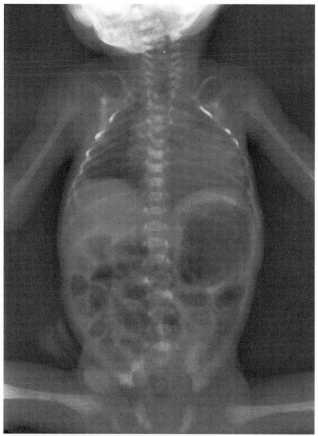

Triploidy (69,XXX)

FIGURE 2–37. Chest radiograph—thin ribs, cardiomegaly due to complex heart disease

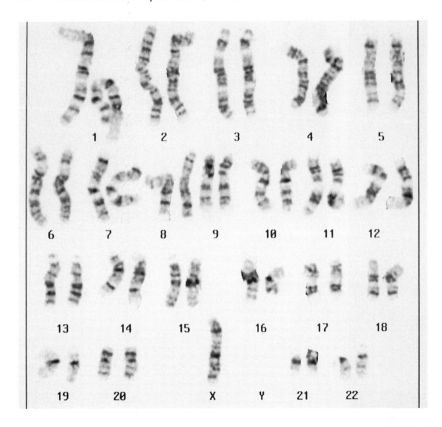

Turner Syndrome

FIGURE 2–39. Karyotype: 45,X

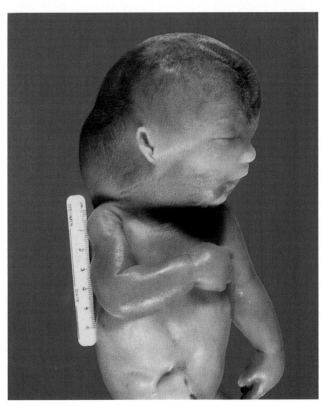

Turner Syndrome

FIGURE 2–40. 24-week fetus, neck edema

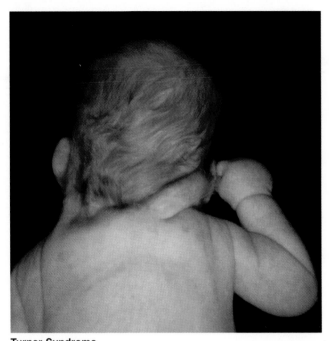

Turner Syndrome

FIGURE 2–41. Webbed neck, low hairline

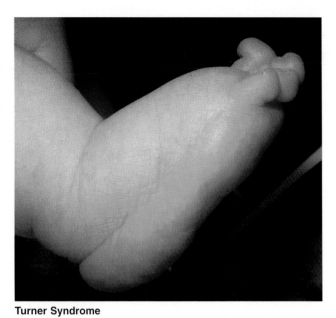

Turner Syndrome

FIGURE 2–43. Pedal lymphedema

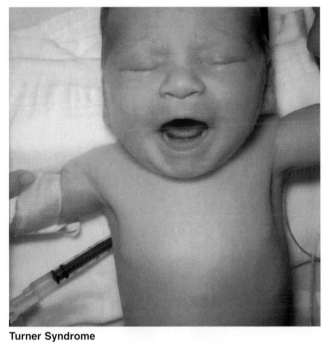

Turner Syndrome

FIGURE 2–42. Broad chest, widespread nipples

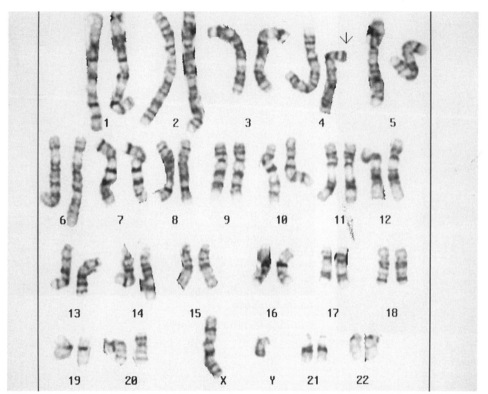

4p− Syndrome

FIGURE 2–44. Karyotype: 46,XY,4p−

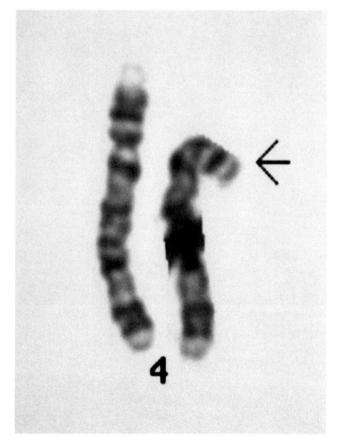

4p− Syndrome

FIGURE 2–45. Banding of chromosome number 4, deletion of short arm

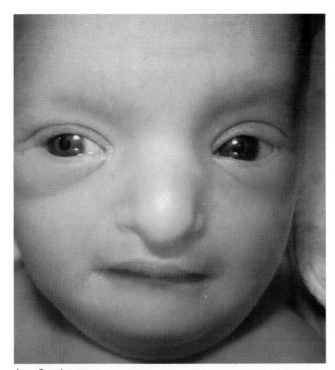

4p− Syndrome

FIGURE 2–46. Beaked nose, hypertelorism

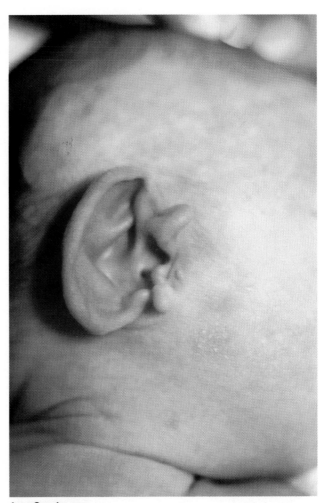

4p− Syndrome

FIGURE 2–48. Redundant ear cartilage

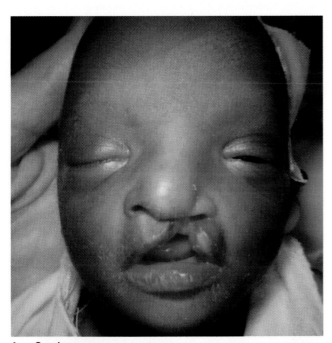

4p− Syndrome

FIGURE 2–47. Cleft lip and palate

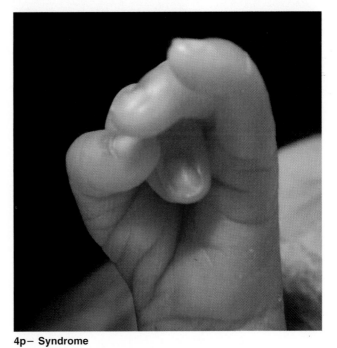

4p− Syndrome

FIGURE 2–49. Hypoplastic hand, overlapped fingers

Nonchromosomal Syndromes

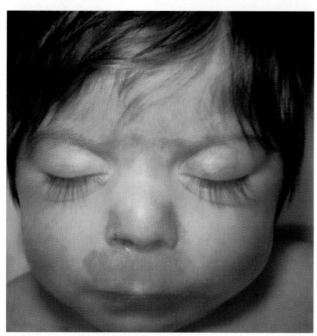

Cornelia de Lange Syndrome

FIGURE 2–50. Face: synophrys

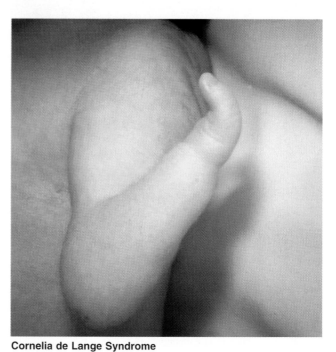

Cornelia de Lange Syndrome

FIGURE 2–52. Hypoplastic arm with monodactyly

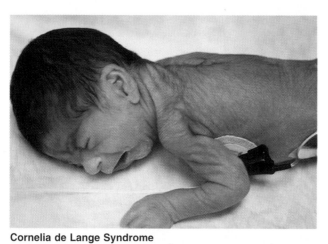

Cornelia de Lange Syndrome

FIGURE 2–51. Body: hirsutism, growth retardation

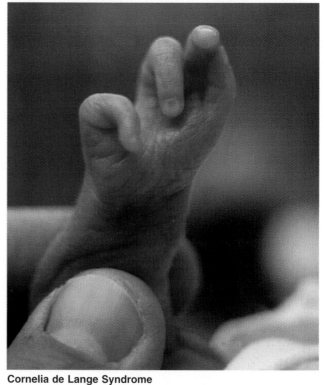

Cornelia de Lange Syndrome

FIGURE 2–53. Cleft, hypoplastic hand with oligodactyly

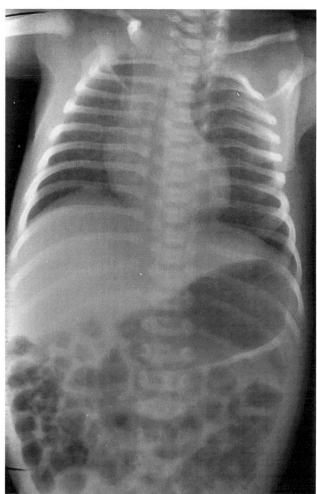

Cornelia de Lange Syndrome

FIGURE 2–54. Chest radiograph: 13 pairs of ribs

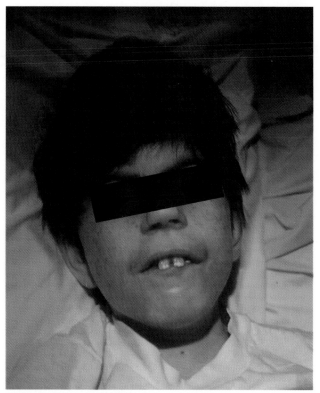

Cornelia de Lange Syndrome

FIGURE 2–55. 6-year-old child—coarse facial features, synophrys

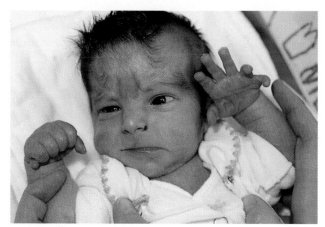

Rubinstein-Taybi Syndrome

FIGURE 2–56. Facial hemangiomas, polydactyly

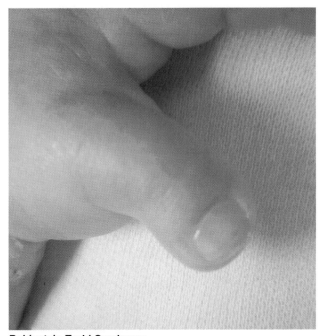

Rubinstein-Taybi Syndrome

FIGURE 2–57. Broad thumb

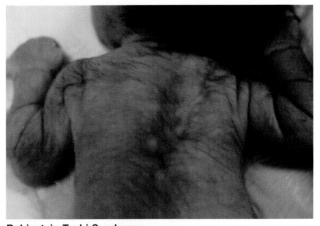

Rubinstein-Taybi Syndrome

FIGURE 2–58. Hirsutism

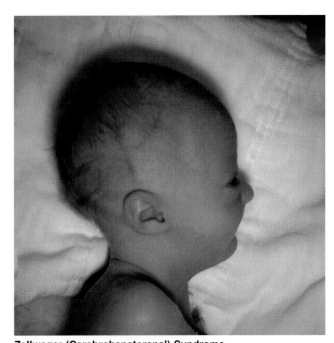

Zellweger (Cerebrohepatorenal) Syndrome

FIGURE 2–59. Profile: globular head, high forehead

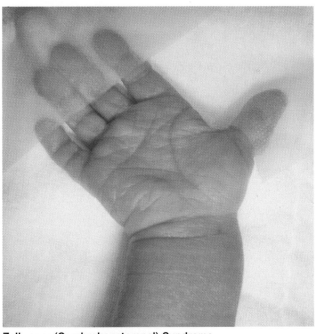

Zellweger (Cerebrohepatorenal) Syndrome

FIGURE 2–60. Complex palmar creases

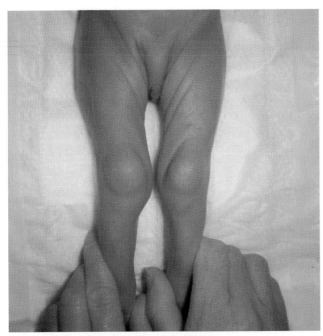

Zellweger (Cerebrohepatorenal) Syndrome

FIGURE 2–61. Prominent knees

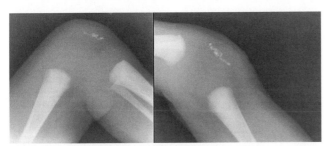

Zellweger (Cerebrohepatorenal) Syndrome

FIGURE 2–62. Radiograph: premature calcification of the patella

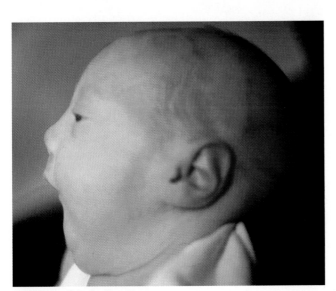

Smith-Lemli-Opitz Syndrome

FIGURE 2–63. Profile: mandibular hypoplasia, sloped forehead, ante-verted nostrils

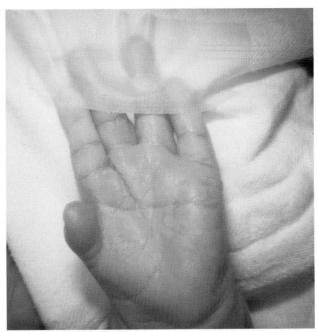

Smith-Lemli-Opitz Syndrome

FIGURE 2–64. Abnormal palmar creases

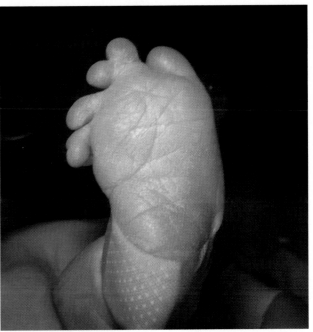

Smith-Lemli-Opitz Syndrome

FIGURE 2–65. Syndactyly of 2nd and 3rd toes

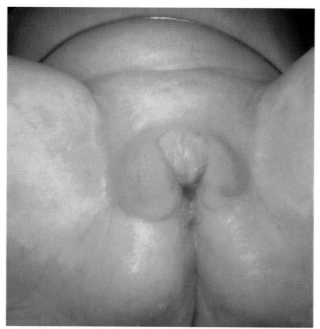

Smith-Lemli-Opitz Syndrome

FIGURE 2–66. Immature, ambiguous genitalia

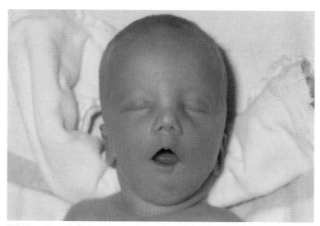

Möbius Syndrome

FIGURE 2–67. Expressionless face

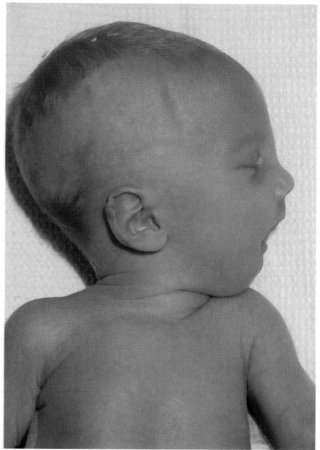

Möbius Syndrome

FIGURE 2–68. Profile: small mandible

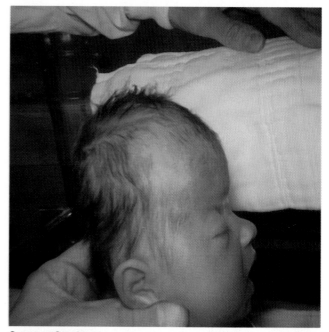

Crouzon Syndrome

FIGURE 2–69. Head profile: skull misshapen due to craniosynostosis

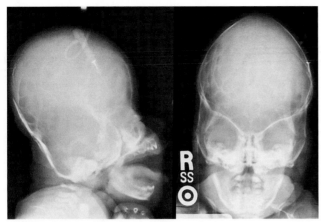

Crouzon Syndrome

FIGURE 2–70. Skull radiograph, AP and lateral views: craniosynostosis

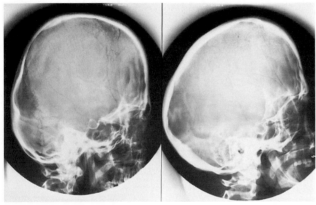

Crouzon Syndrome

FIGURE 2–71. Radiograph: skull profiles of the preceding infant's mother and grandmother

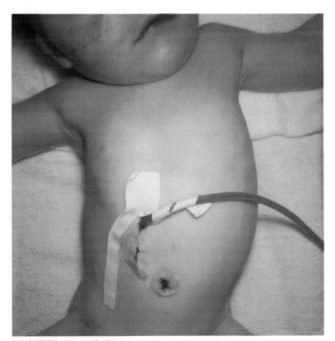

VACTERL Association

FIGURE 2–72. Trunk curvature due to scoliosis

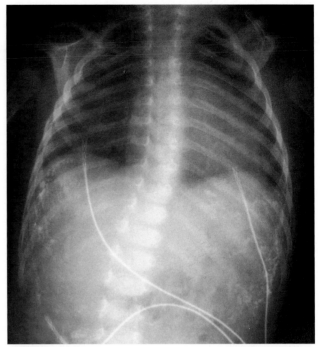

VACTERL Association

FIGURE 2–73. Radiograph: rib malformations, tracheoesophageal fistula

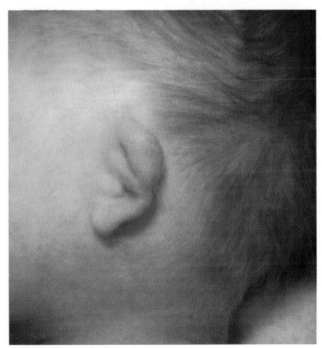

VACTERL Association

FIGURE 2–74. Hypoplastic pinna

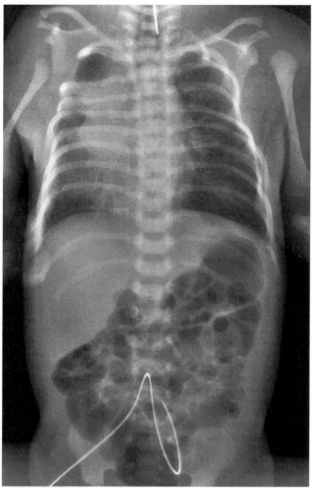

VACTERL Association

FIGURE 2–75. Radiograph: complex thoracic vertebral anomalies, tracheoesophageal fistula

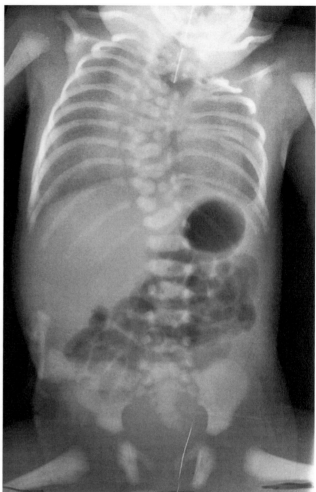

VACTERL Association

FIGURE 2–76. Radiograph: multiple vertebral anomalies, tracheoesophageal fistula, cardiomegaly due to complex congenital heart disease

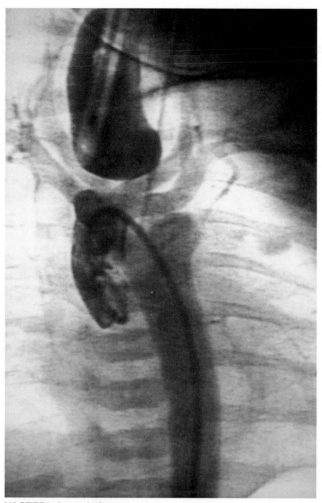

VACTERL Association

FIGURE 2–77. Aortic arteriogram: thoracic vascular ring, contrast in esophageal pouch

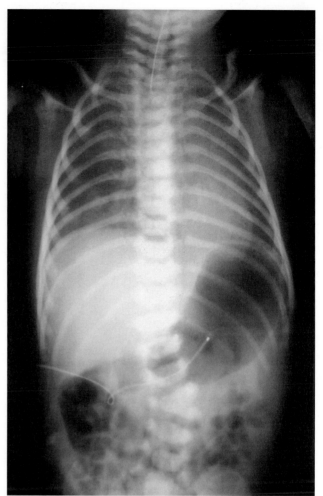

VACTERL Association

FIGURE 2–78. Radiograph: lumbar vertebral anomalies

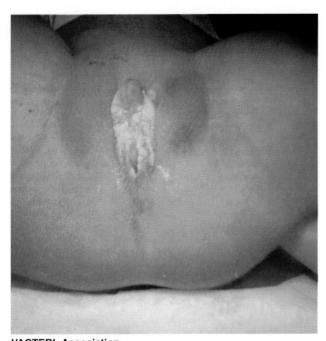

VACTERL Association

FIGURE 2–79. Anal atresia

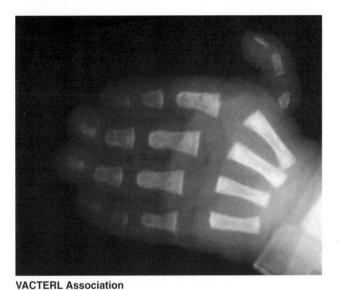

VACTERL Association

FIGURE 2–80. Radiograph: hypoplastic thumb

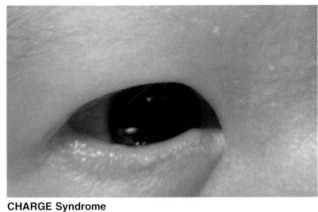

CHARGE Syndrome

FIGURE 2–81. Coloboma

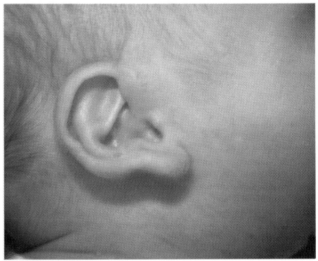

CHARGE Syndrome

FIGURE 2–82. Pinna posteriorly rotated

SELECTED REFERENCES

Graham JM. (1990) Fetal dysmorphology. Clin Perinatol 17:3.
Jones KL. (1997) Smith's Recognizable Patterns of Human Malformation, 5th ed. Philadelphia, WB Saunders.
Moore KL and Persaud TVN. (1998) The Developing Human, 6th ed. Philadelphia, WB Saunders.
Polin RA and Fox WW. (1998) Fetal and Neonatal Physiology, 2nd ed. Philadelphia, WB Saunders, Chapters 2–4.
Taeusch HW and Ballard RA. (1998) Avery's Diseases of the Newborn, 7th ed. Philadelphia, WB Saunders, Chapters 17-27.
Workman ML, Kenner C, and Hilse MA. Human genetics. In Kenner C, Brueggemeyer A, and Gunderson LP, Eds. (1993) Comprehensive Neonatal Nursing. Philadelphia, WB Saunders.

3 Perinatal Infections

The fetus and newborn infant are at great risk of infection from a wide variety of organisms (Table 3-1). The following information will give a brief look at the problems with the immune system as well as clinical correlates of the various infections.

The defense of the fetus and neonate against infection can be divided into those factors contributed by the mother and those by the infant. The basement membranes of the placenta and a long, occluded cervix provide a physical barrier to infectious agents. These can be breached by a number of organisms (Table 3-2; see p. 74). Active transport of immunoglobulin G (IgG) across the placenta becomes clinically significant only after approximately 18 to 20 weeks of gestation. By the time of delivery, the concentration of IgG in infants is higher than that in the mothers. Only trace amounts of the other immunoglobulins reach the fetus.

The fetal defense against infection is poor but slowly increases throughout gestation. The preterm newborn's physical barriers to infection are insufficient. The very thin, poorly keratinized skin is prone to breakdown that permits invasion from infectious agents. There is much controversy over the circulating phagocytic cells. In vitro, when adult sera are added, the neutrophils exhibit near-normal phagocytic function. However, in their usual environment, circulating neutrophils have decreased chemotaxis and decreased phagocytosis. Circulating monocytes and tissue macrophages in the skin, intestine, and liver also are less effective than those of adults.

The ability to kill intracellular organisms is normal, but an insufficient storage pool of neutrophils allows the newborn infant to be overwhelmed by infections more easily than an older child. Although the T-cell and B-cell lymphocytes are generally quiescent in utero, if challenged they can respond and produce immunoglobulins and cytokines.

TABLE 3-1

		TIMING OF INFECTION	
	PRENATAL (TRANSPLACENTAL)	PERINATAL	POSTNATAL
BACTERIAL	*Listeria*	Group B streptococcus *Escherichia coli* *Listeria*	Many gram-negative bacteria Late-onset Group B streptococcus *Staphylococcus aureus* *S. epidermidis* Tetanus Tuberculosis
VIRAL	Rubella Cytomegalovirus HIV	HIV Cytomegalovirus Hepatitis B Varicella Herpes simplex Echovirus Coxsackievirus	Herpes simplex Coxsackievirus Hepatitis B
OTHER	Toxoplasmosis Syphilis Malaria	Verruca: vulgaris or acuminata	*Candida*

HIV, human immunodeficiency virus

55

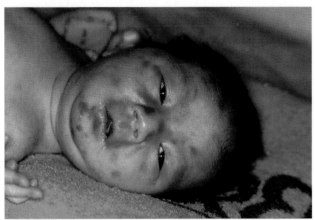

Rubella

FIGURE 3–1. "Blueberry muffin" multiple purpura due to thrombocytopenia and extramedullary hematopoiesis

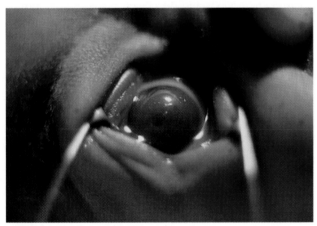

Rubella

FIGURE 3–2. Glaucoma and iritis

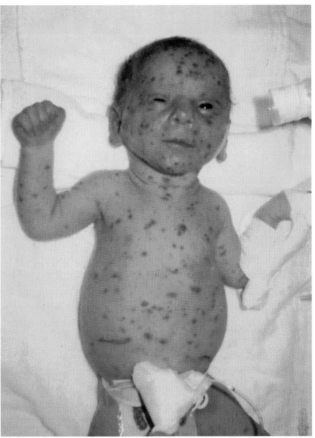

Cytomegalovirus (CMV)

FIGURE 3–3. Hepatosplenomegaly, jaundice

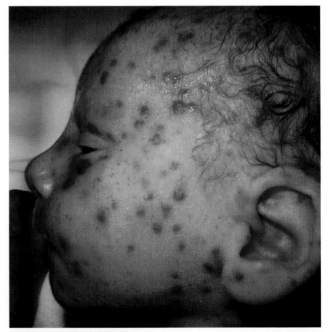

Cytomegalovirus (CMV)

FIGURE 3–4. Petechiae and purpura

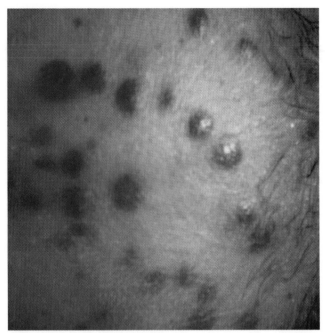

Cytomegalovirus (CMV)

FIGURE 3–5. Dermal extramedullary hematopoiesis

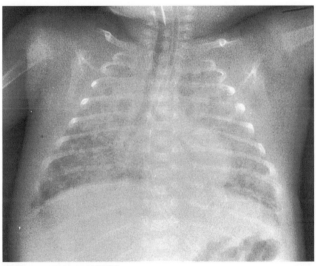

Cytomegalovirus (CMV)

FIGURE 3–6. Chest radiograph: diffuse CMV pneumonia

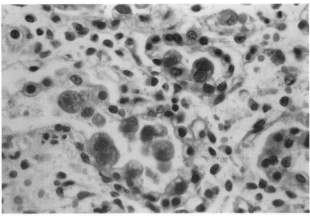

Cytomegalovirus (CMV)

FIGURE 3–7. CMV inclusions in postmortem lung

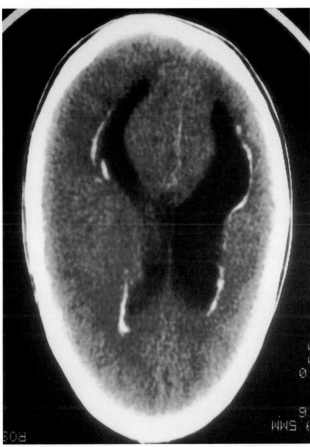

Cytomegalovirus (CMV)

FIGURE 3–8. Cranial CT scan—hydrocephalus, periventricular calcification

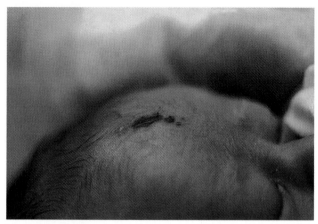

Herpes (Type II)

FIGURE 3–9. Scalp herpes, vertex delivery

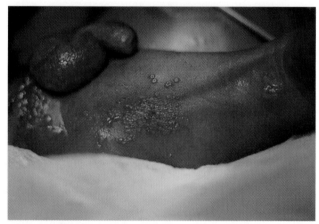

Herpes (Type II)

FIGURE 3–10. Perineal herpes, breech delivery

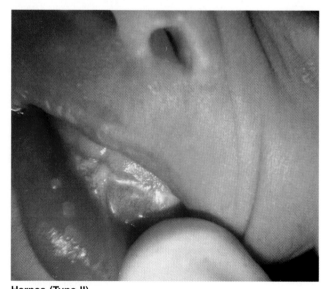

Herpes (Type II)

FIGURE 3–11. Lip herpes, from maternal herpes breast lesions

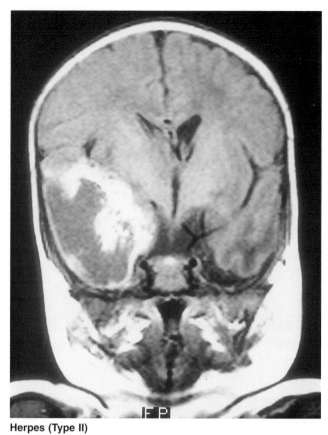

Herpes (Type II)

FIGURE 3–12. MRI—localized herpes encephalitis of the parietal lobe

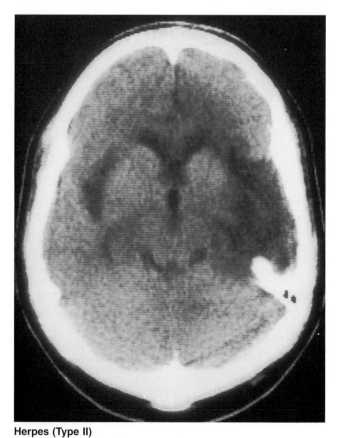

Herpes (Type II)

FIGURE 3–13. CT scan—diffuse encephalitis

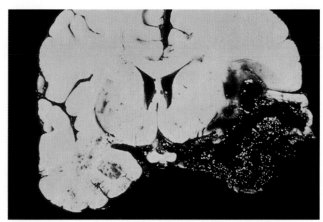

Herpes (Type II)

FIGURE 3–14. Cross-section of necrotic temporal lobe

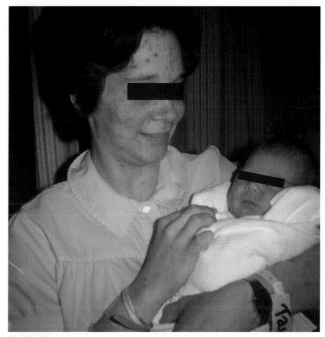

Varicella

FIGURE 3–15. Maternal varicella, healthy baby

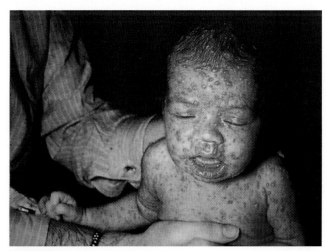

Varicella

FIGURE 3–16. Acute neonatal varicella

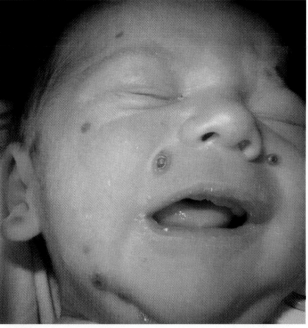

Varicella

FIGURE 3–17. Crusting lesions

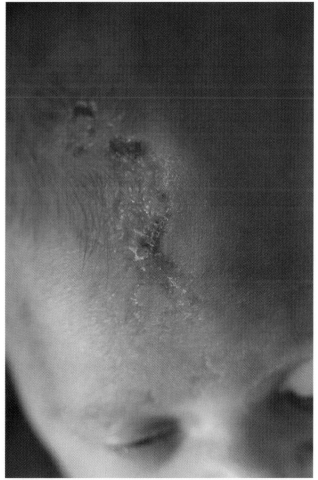

Varicella

FIGURE 3–18. Cicatricial scalp lesions of congenital varicella

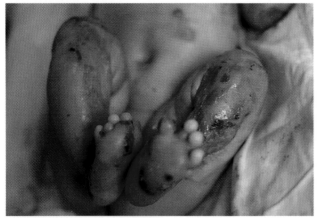

Varicella

FIGURE 3–19. Cicatricial skin lesions and limb hypoplasia

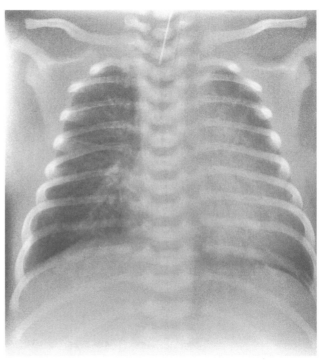

Enterovirus

FIGURE 3–21. Radiograph: enteroviral myocarditis

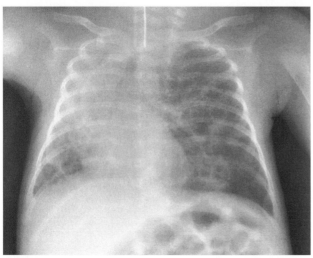

Papillomavirus

FIGURE 3–20. Radiograph: atelectasis due to airway warts

BACTERIA

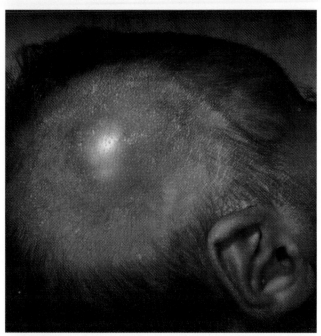

Gonorrhea

FIGURE 3–22. Scalp abscess

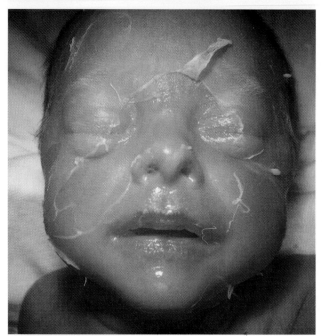

Staphylococcus aureus

FIGURE 3–24. Scalded skin syndrome of face

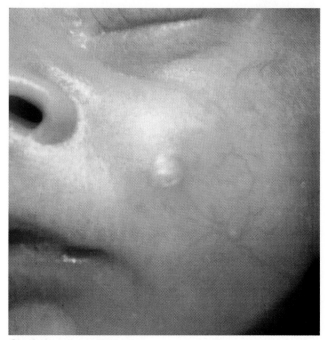

Staphylococcus aureus

FIGURE 3–23. Facial pustule

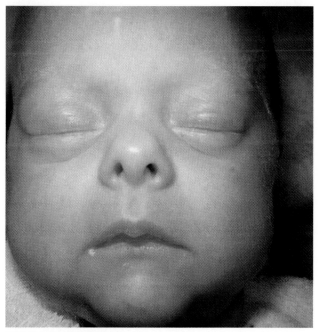

Staphylococcus aureus

FIGURE 3–25. Scalded skin syndrome, healed

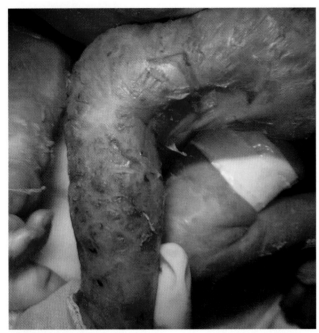

Staphylococcus aureus

FIGURE 3–26. Scalded skin syndrome of leg

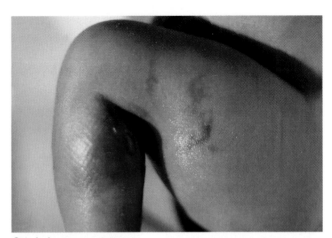

Staphylococcus aureus

FIGURE 3–28. Thigh abscess

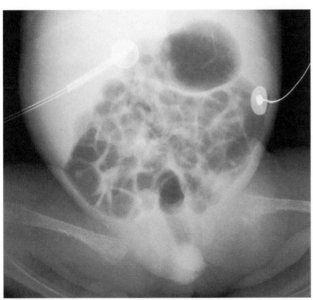

Staphylococcus aureus

FIGURE 3–27. Radiograph: staphylococcal septic arthritis and osteomyelitis of left hip

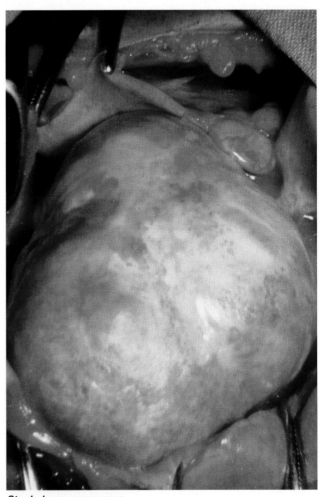

Staphylococcus aureus

FIGURE 3–29. Pericarditis

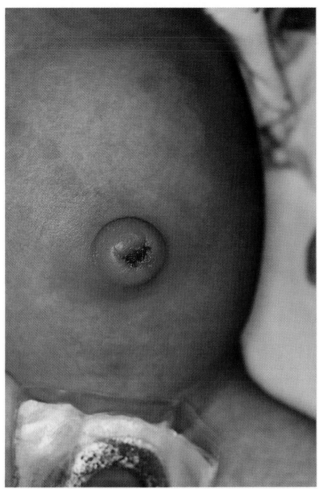

Staphylococcus aureus

FIGURE 3–30. Omphalitis

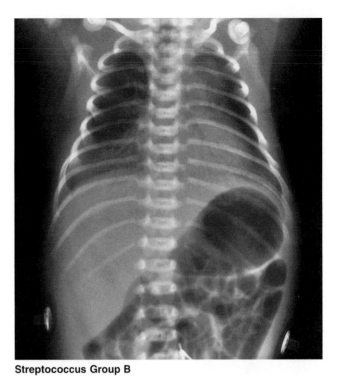

Streptococcus Group B

FIGURE 3–32. Chest radiograph: pneumonia, early respiratory distress

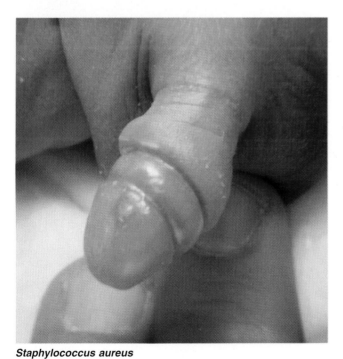

Staphylococcus aureus

FIGURE 3–31. Infected penis following circumcision

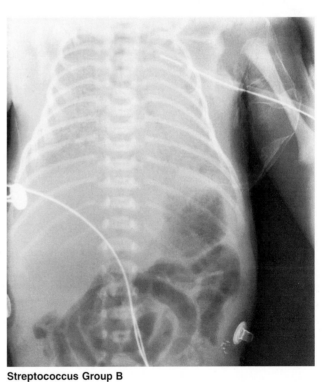

Streptococcus Group B

FIGURE 3–33. Chest radiograph: pneumonia, rapid consolidation over 3 hours

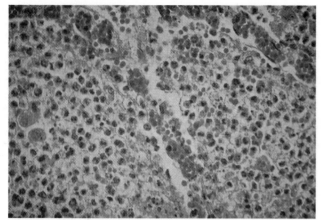

Streptococcus Group B

FIGURE 3–34. Pathology: lobar pneumonia

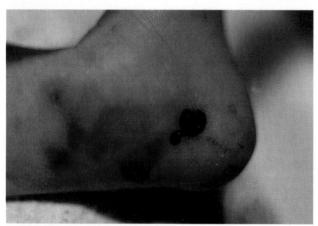

Streptococcus Group B

FIGURE 3–35. Cellulitis of the site of an IV infiltrate

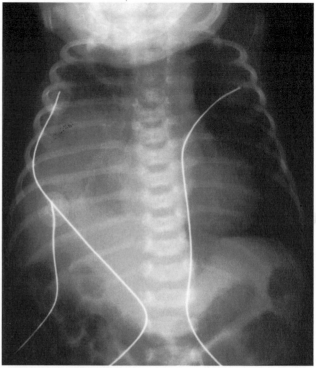

Streptococcus Group B

FIGURE 3–36. Chest radiograph: right lower lobe pneumonia causing paralysis of the right hemidiaphragm

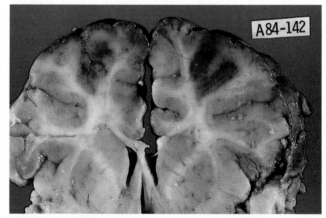

Streptococcus Group B

FIGURE 3–37. *Haemophilus influenzae* meningitis with brain infarction

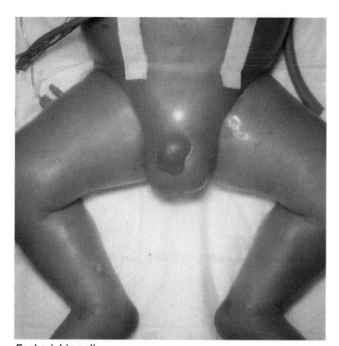

Escherichia coli

FIGURE 3–38. Sclerema—systemic sepsis

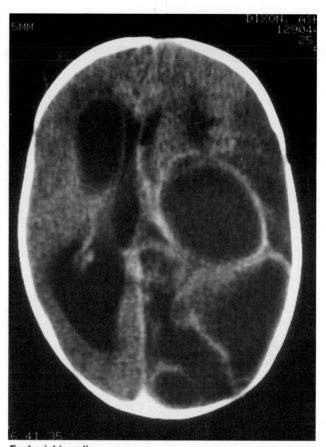

Escherichia coli

FIGURE 3–40. CT scan: progressive brain destruction

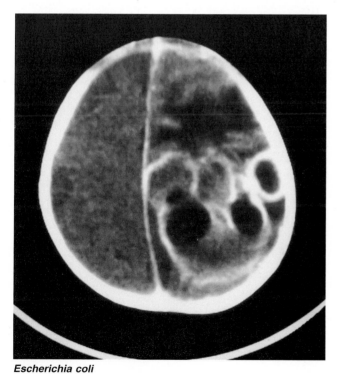

Escherichia coli

FIGURE 3–39. CT scan: loculated brain abscess

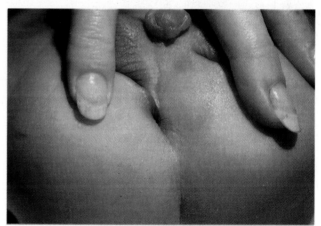

Escherichia coli

FIGURE 3–41. Perineal abscess

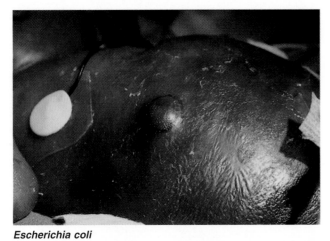

Escherichia coli

FIGURE 3–42. Peritonitis

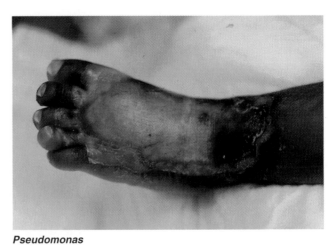

Pseudomonas

FIGURE 3–44. Foot necrosis from systemic infection

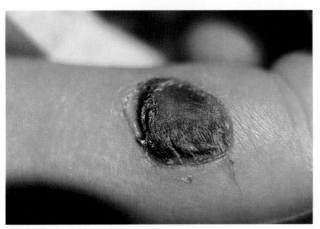

Pseudomonas

FIGURE 3–43. Necrosis from localized infection—ecthyma gangrenosum

FUNGI

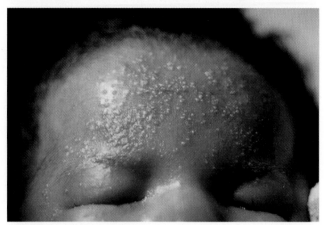

Candida

FIGURE 3–45. Cutaneous candidiasis of the forehead at birth

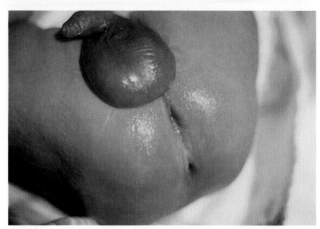

Candida

FIGURE 3–48. Diaper rash

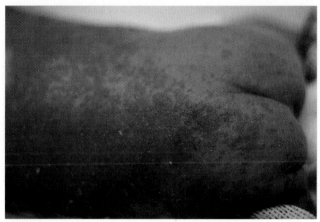

Candida

FIGURE 3–46. Cutaneous candidiasis of the back

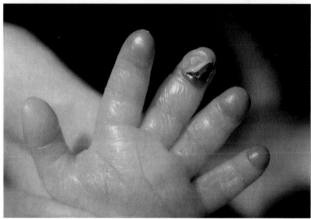

Candida

FIGURE 3–49. Systemic candidiasis, necrosis of fingertips

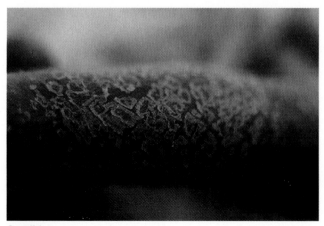

Candida

FIGURE 3–47. Resolving, scaling skin

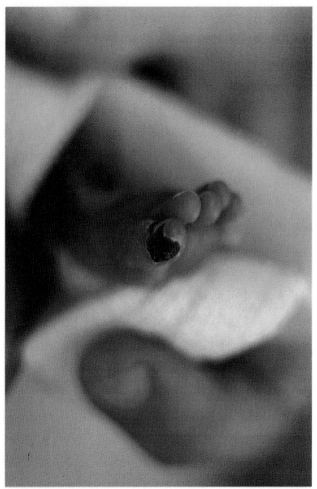

Candida

FIGURE 3–50. Toe necrosis from candidiasis

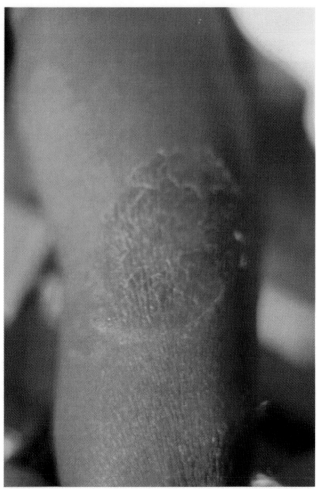

Tinea

FIGURE 3–51. Tinea corporis of leg

PROTOZOA

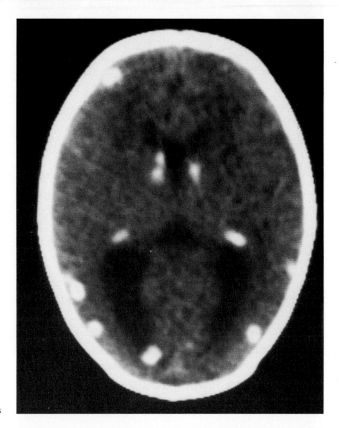

Toxoplasmosis

FIGURE 3–52. Scattered cerebral calcifications

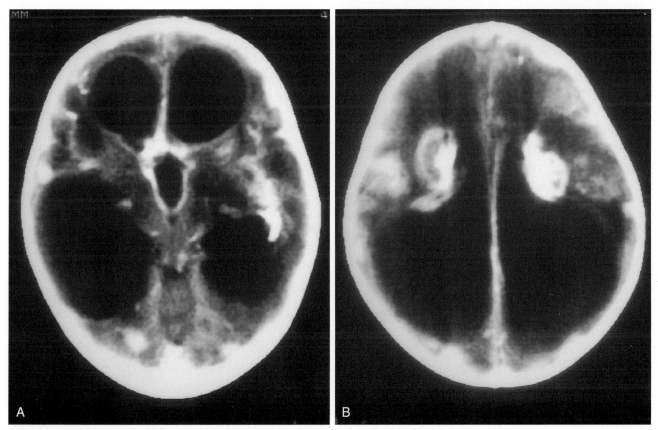

Twins with Severe Toxoplasmosis of the Brain

FIGURE 3–53. Twin A: two views of severe hydrocephalus

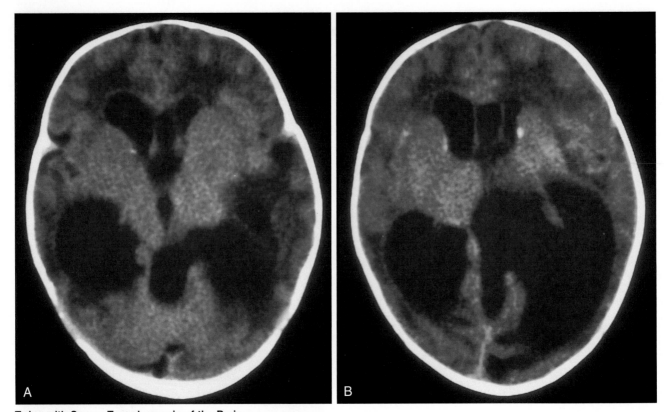

Twins with Severe Toxoplasmosis of the Brain

FIGURE 3–54. Twin B: two views of infarct and necrosis of the brain

SYPHILIS

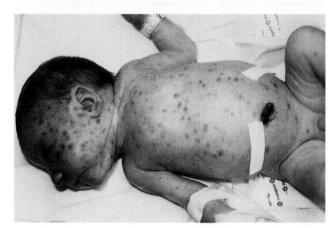

FIGURE 3–55. Diffuse purpura

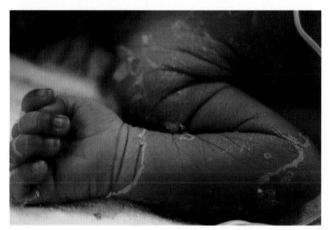

FIGURE 3–56. Scaling rash

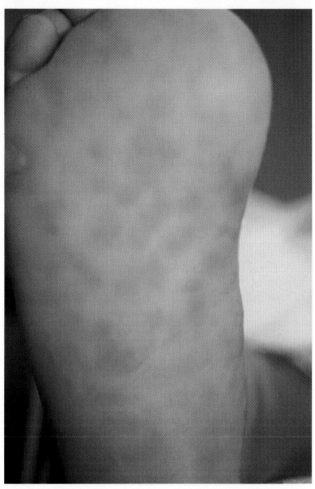

FIGURE 3–57. Sole of foot—multiple erythematous macules

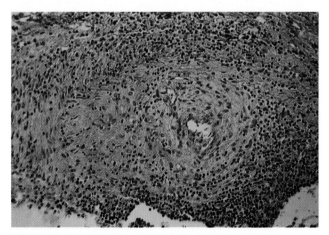

FIGURE 3–58. Histology: syphilitic endarteritis

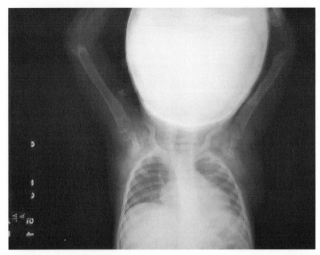

FIGURE 3–59. Chest radiograph: periostitis of ribs and long bones

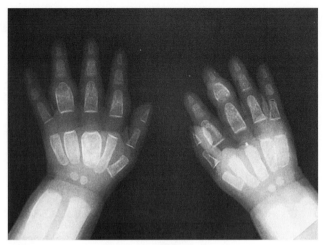

FIGURE 3–61. Hand radiograph: syphilitic dactylitis

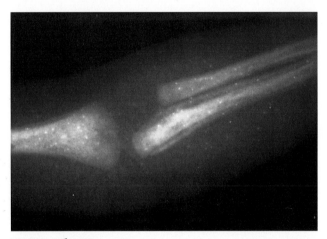

FIGURE 3–60. Elbow radiograph: periostitis

PNEUMOCYSTIS

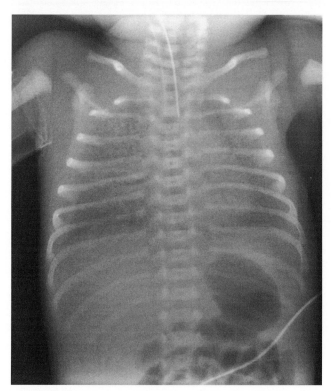

FIGURE 3–62. Chest radiograph: diffuse interstitial pneumonia

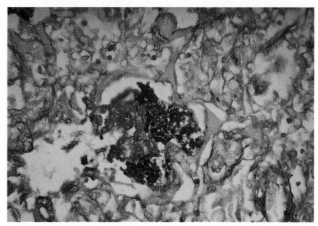

FIGURE 3–63. Lung histology: silver stain of the organism

TABLE 3-2

ORGAN SYSTEM–SPECIFIC BACTERIAL INFECTIONS

INFECTION	ORGANISM	CLINICAL FINDINGS
Meningitis	Group B streptococcus, *Escherichia coli* *Listeria* Gram-negative bacteria	Often presents as sepsis with lethargy, poor tone, poor feeding; classic stiff neck often absent. *Listeria* and Group B streptococcus may have a late-onset, less fulminant course
Pneumonia	Initially most likely Group B streptococcus or *E. coli.* Later nosocomial pneumonias of other gram-negatives, *Staphylococcus aureus,* and *Candida*	Respiratory distress that can rapidly deteriorate into fulminant sepsis syndrome
Ophthalmologic	Initially chemical conjunctivitis. *Neisseria* and chlamydia most common. *Staphylococcus, streptococcus,* and *Pseudomonas* also seen	Purulent drainage persisting past the 1–2 days seen with chemical conjunctivitis; the cornea may be involved
Septic arthritis and osteomyelitis	*S. aureus,* occasionally Group A or Group B streptococcus	Usually only local swelling; tenderness often without fever or systemic signs until much later
Skin and mucous membranes	*S. aureus,* Group A streptococcus, *Pseudomonas, Candida,* herpes	Localized abscess under former scalp electrode sites, mucosal infections by *Candida,* life-threatening disseminated by Group B streptococcus, *Pseudomonas*

SELECTED REFERENCES

Lott JW and Kenner C. Assessment and management of immunologic dysfunction. *In* Kenner C, Brueggemeyer A, and Gunderson LP, Eds. (1993) Comprehensive Neonatal Nursing. Philadelphia, WB Saunders.

Polin RA and Fox WW. (1998) Fetal and Neonatal Physiology. Philadelphia, WB Saunders, Chapters 174–179.

Stoll BJ and Weismen LE. (1997) Perinatal infections. Clin Perinatol 24:1.

Taeusch HW and Ballard RA. (19981) Avery's Diseases of the Newborn. Philadelphia, WB Saunders, Chapters 41–47.

4 Respiratory

Knowledge about the embryologic formation of the lung and its surrounding tissues is of great advantage when trying to understand the pathophysiology of neonatal pulmonary disease. Following is a very brief description of early lung formation and several tables describing lung development and some of the more common structural and functional abnormalities (Tables 4–1 and 4–2).

At approximately 22 to 26 days of gestation, a small outpouching occurs on the ventral side of the primitive foregut. These endodermally derived cells push into a group of mesodermal cells. The endodermal cells differentiate to form all of the air passages and alveoli, whereas the mesodermal cells are the earliest precursors of connective tissue and blood vessels. Over the next 4 weeks, there is a steady expansion of both the support structures and the dividing, expanding airways that begin to form the early lung.

From the 8th to 16th week of gestation, the airways branch aggressively until the total adult complement of air passages is reached. At the same time, the two arterial systems, one from the aorta and one from the pulmonary artery, take form and grow extensively along with the air passages. Although the muscular cartilage and lymphatic and bronchial glandular tissues do not develop as soon as the airways and blood vessels do, by the end of the 14th week all have a significant presence in the early lung.

The 17th to 24th weeks are characterized by a marked increase in the number of bronchioles and alveoli. Although branching of the pulmonary arteries has

TABLE 4–1

STAGES OF LUNG DEVELOPMENT	
POSTCONCEPTUAL AGE (Wk)	MAJOR EVENTS
3–7	Lung budding and epithelium mesenchymal interaction
8–16	Completion of airway division; cartilage and smooth muscle development
17–27	Capillary development, alveolar development; Types I and II pneumocytes
28–35	Thinning of epithelial cells; thinning of the blood vessel walls; terminal saccular formation
>36	Appearance of true alveoli and alveolar septation

TABLE 4–2

CONGENITAL PULMONARY MALFORMATIONS			
ABNORMALITY	TIMING	PATHOLOGY	EPIDEMIOLOGY
Cystic adenomatous malformation	Variable	Type I large cyst	Most common, approximately 50%
		Type II smaller cyst	Often associated with anomalies
		Type III cyst <0.5 cm	Constitutes only 5%
Pulmonary sequestration	<8 wk	Extrapulmonary	Left lung > right lung; male extrapulmonary pathology has frequent incidence of concomitant congenital anomaly
		Intrapulmonary	Rare congenital anomaly; left > right; male > female
Lobar emphysema	Variable	Marked overdistention of alveoli; obstruction found in 25%	Usually upper lobes; male > female
Bronchogenic cyst	By 16th wk	Early cyst found in mediastinum; later cyst formation in peripheral parenchymal cysts	Uncommon
Diaphragmatic hernia	Often <16 wk	Incomplete closure of muscular diaphragm with abdominal dysraphism compromising lung development and function	1 in 2000 to 1 in 4000

TABLE 4-3

COMMON FORMS OF NEONATAL RESPIRATORY DISTRESS

ABNORMALITY	PATHOLOGY	CLINICAL MANIFESTATIONS
Meconium aspiration	Mechanical plugging, chemical irritant effect, fatty acid stripping of surfactant	Airway plugging, alveolar collapse, arteriovenous mismatching
Pneumonia	Wide range of neonatal fetally acquired or neonatal viral and bacterial infections	Spectrum from asymptomatic to severe respiratory failure in the first minutes of life
Transient tachypnea (retained lung fluid)	Imbalance in pulmonary fluid production and ability of lung to clear it; possibly ion pump defect	Decreased compliance and oxygenation resulting in increased respiratory effort and rate
Respiratory distress syndrome	Surfactant insufficiency and associated vascular and interstitial effects	Hypoxia, hypercapnia, right to left shunting—pulmonary and cardiac
Persistent pulmonary hypertension	Abnormal vascular tone or thickened vascular structure resulting in marked increased resistance in blood flow through the lung	Intrapulmonary, intracardiac shunting leads to a cycle of worsening hypoxia and acidosis

stopped, there is continued growth in length and thinning of the vessel walls in preparation for gas exchange. The final 16 weeks of pulmonary development include the proliferation and maturation of Type I and Type II pneumocytes, a marked increase in alveoli, and concomitant growth in alveolar capillaries.

Given the complex development of the lung, congenital structural abnormalities and acquired functional abnormalities have markedly different clinical presentations (Table 4-3).

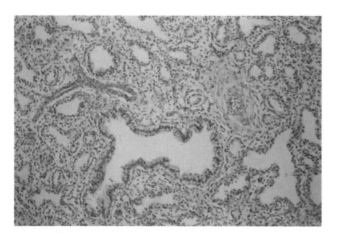

FIGURE 4-1. Histology: dense, poorly differentiated lung of a 500-gm fetus

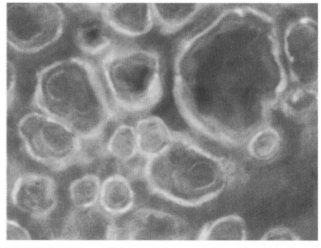

FIGURE 4-2. Normal variation of shape and size of alveoli at the surface of the lung

NORMAL CHEST RADIOGRAPHS

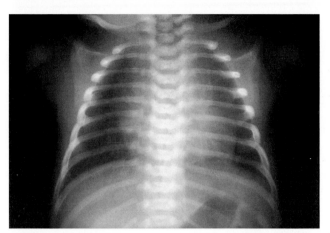

FIGURE 4-3. Anteroposterior radiograph of a normal lung

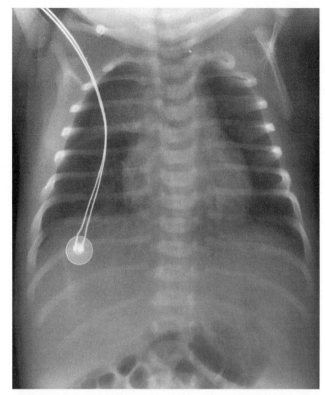

FIGURE 4-4. Anteroposterior radiograph of a well-inflated normal lung with an asymmetric thymus

PULMONARY HYPOPLASIA

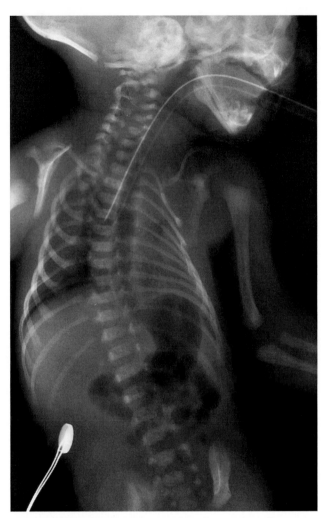

FIGURE 4–5. Primary hypoplasia resulting from prolonged amniotic fluid leak and severe oligohydramnios

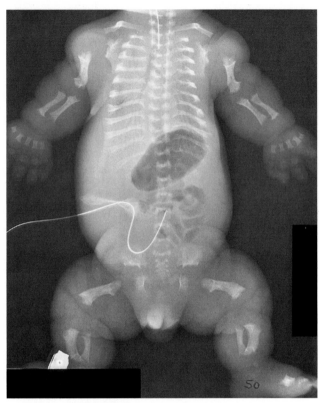

FIGURE 4–7. Asphyxiating thoracic dystrophy

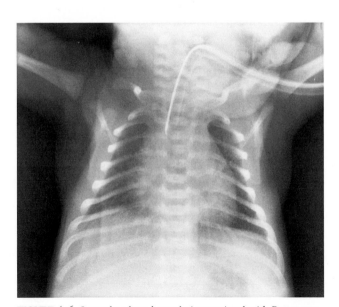

FIGURE 4–6. Secondary lung hypoplasia associated with Potter syndrome

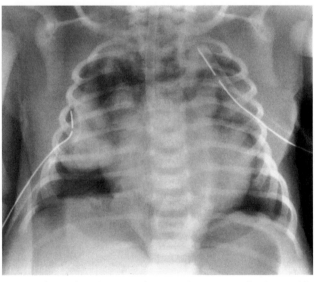

FIGURE 4–8. Bilateral pneumothorax and pneumomediastinum with severe pulmonary hypoplasia

TRANSIENT TACHYPNEA (RETAINED LUNG FLUID)

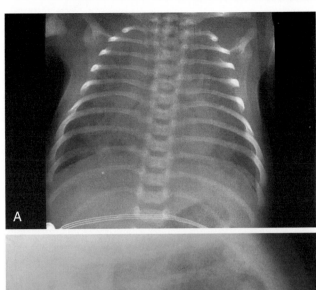

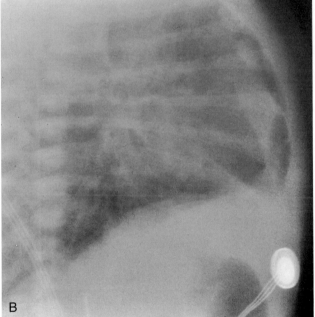

FIGURE 4–9. A, Anteroposterior radiograph at birth; perihilar fluid density. B, Lateral view at birth; major and minor fissures are prominent.

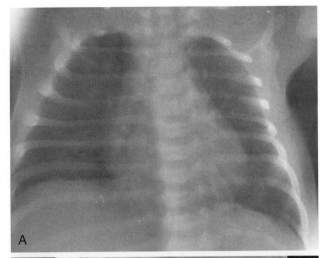

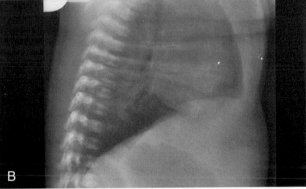

FIGURE 4–10. A, Anteroposterior radiograph at 36 hours, clear lung fields. B, Lateral view at 36 hours, clear lungs

SURFACTANT DEFICIENCY—HYALINE MEMBRANE DISEASE

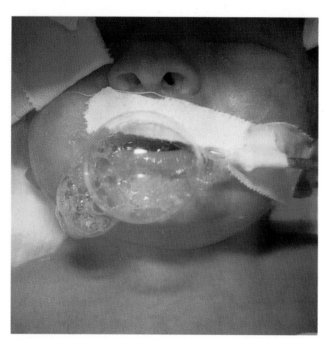

FIGURE 4–11. "Bubbles" of surfactant

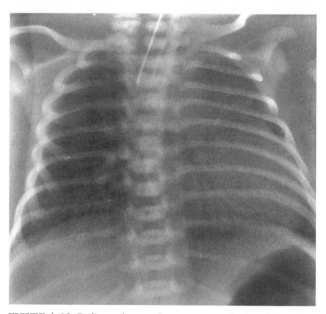

FIGURE 4–12. Radiograph: granular appearance due to microatelectasis with air bronchograms

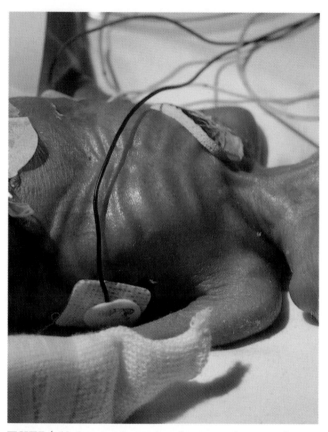

FIGURE 4–13. Intercostal retractions due to poor lung compliance

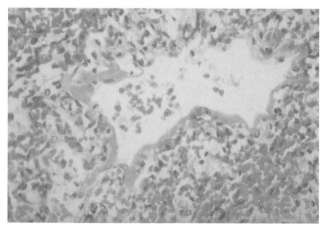

FIGURE 4–14. Histology: alveolar collapse, hyaline membranes

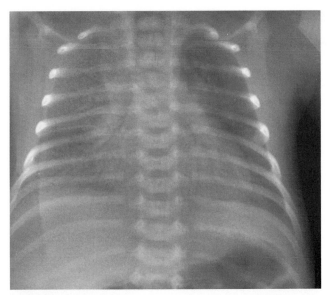

FIGURE 4–15. Radiograph of asymmetric surfactant deficiency

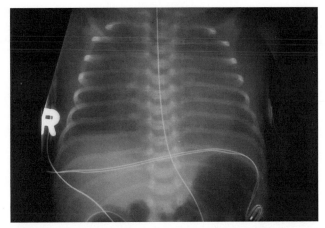

FIGURE 4–17. Radiograph: after surfactant replacement therapy

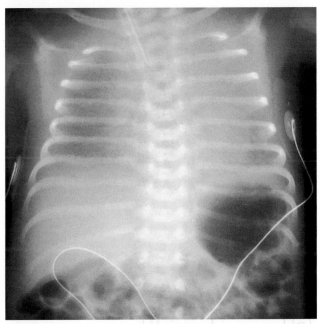

FIGURE 4–16. Radiograph: before surfactant replacement therapy

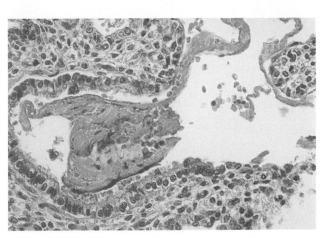

FIGURE 4–18. Histology after surfactant replacement therapy: congealed surfactant in a small airway

MECONIUM ASPIRATION SYNDROME

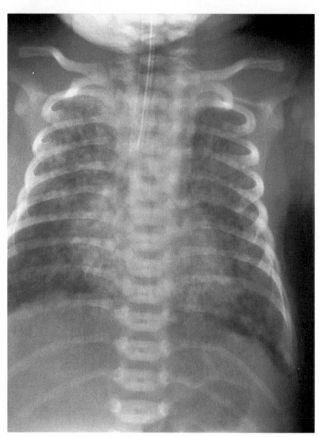

FIGURE 4–19. Air trapping—hyperexpansion from airway obstruction

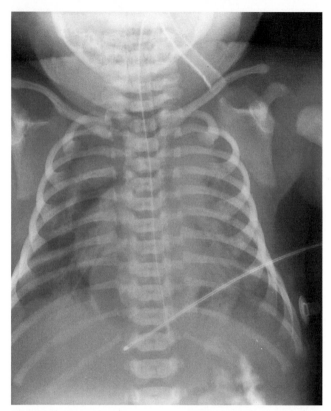

FIGURE 4–20. Acute atelectasis due to surfactant inactivation

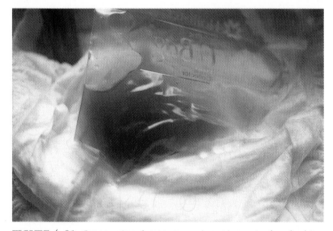

FIGURE 4–21. Green urine due to meconium pigments absorbed in the lung within 12 hours of aspiration

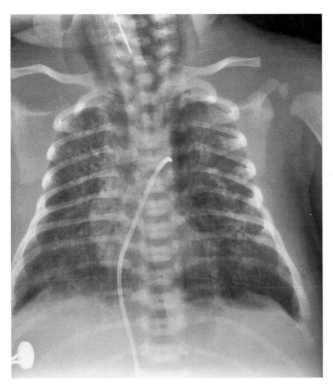

FIGURE 4–22. Pneumomediastinum from gas trapping and airway leak

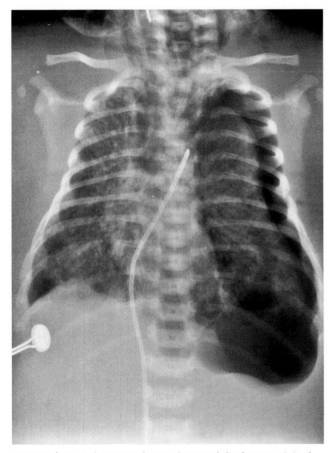

FIGURE 4–23. Left pneumothorax: depressed diaphragm; minimal mediastinal shift due to noncompliant lungs

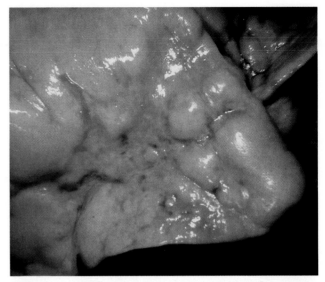

FIGURE 4–24. Lung surface: atelectasis from surfactant deficiency

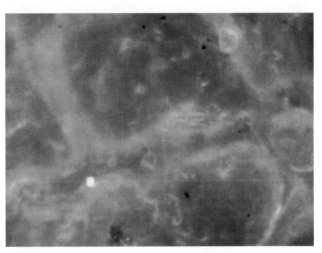

FIGURE 4–25. Surface alveoli, hyperexpanded from partial airway obstruction

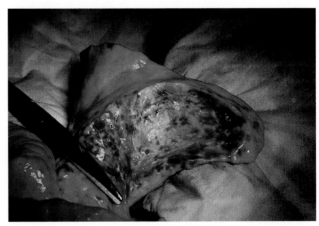

FIGURE 4–26. Lung cross-section demonstrating distal distribution of meconium

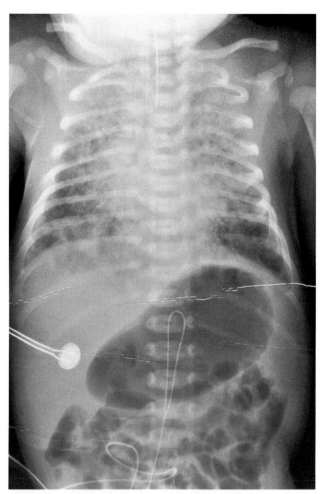

FIGURE 4–27. Diffuse chemical pneumonitis from constituents of meconium

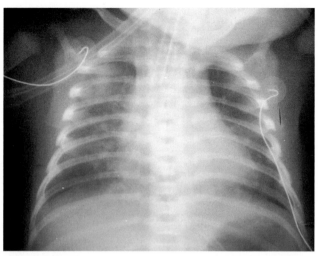

FIGURE 4–28. Amniotic fluid aspiration

PROGRESSION FROM ACUTE SURFACTANT DEFICIENCY TO BRONCHOPULMONARY DYSPLASIA

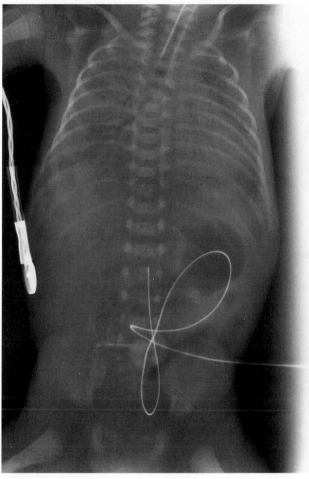

FIGURE 4–29. Birth: early surfactant deficiency

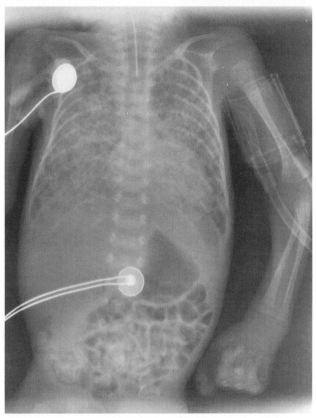

FIGURE 4–30. 1 month: interspersed atelectasis and hyperinflation

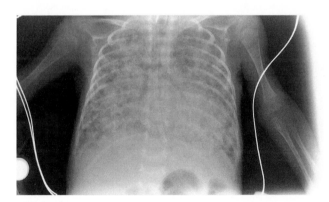

FIGURE 4–31. 2 months: asymmetric progressive inflammation, microcysts

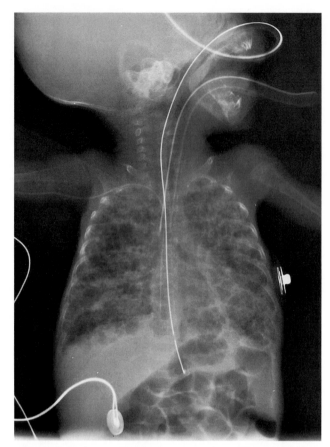

FIGURE 4-32. 3 months: enlarging cysts, diffuse inflammation

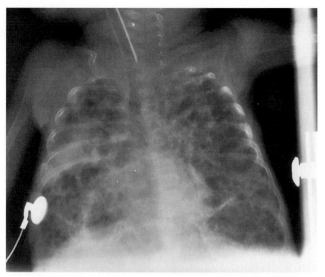

FIGURE 4-33. 4 months: fibrosis, adhesions, cysts of varying size, atelectasis

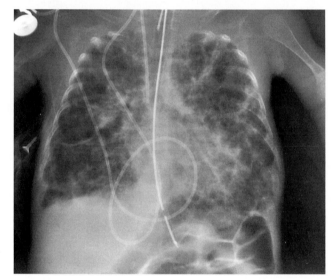

FIGURE 4-34. 5 months: hyperexpansion, air trapping, migrating atelectasis

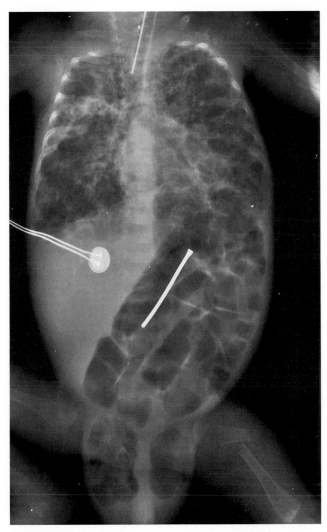

FIGURE 4–35. 6 months: end stage, premortem "stiff" lungs with cor pulmonale

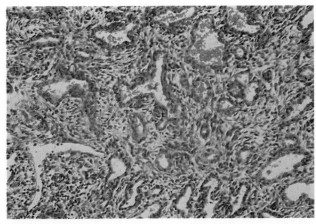

FIGURE 4–36. Pulmonary histology of bronchopulmonary dysplasia: diffuse connective tissue (blue), inflammation, and little alveolar surface area

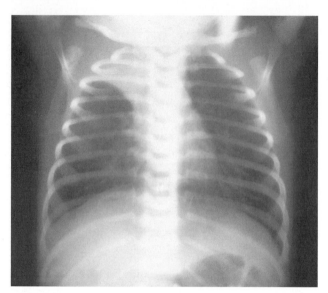

FIGURE 4–37. Right upper lobe with upward bowing of minor fissure

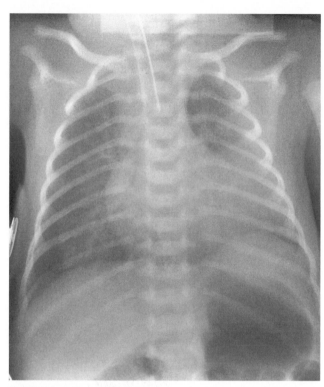

FIGURE 4–39. Lingual atelectasis—loss of the left heart border with elevated left diaphragm

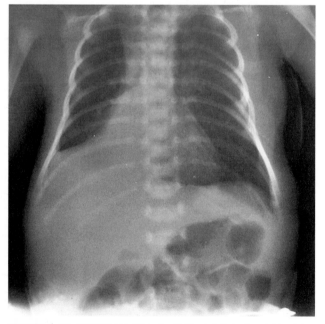

FIGURE 4–38. Right lower lobe, mediastinal shift to the right, and the dome of the right diaphragm obscured

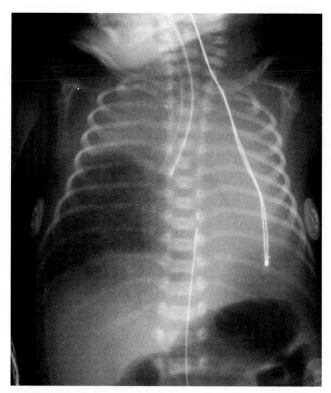

FIGURE 4–40. Atelectasis of the left lung and right upper lobe due to right main stem intubation

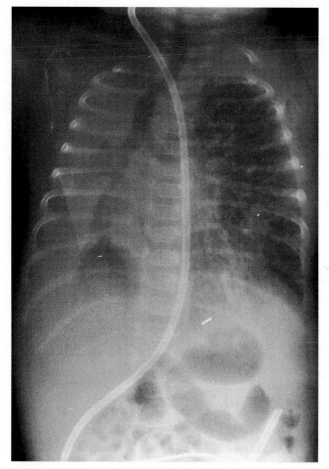

FIGURE 4–41. Postextubation atelectasis of right lung, trachea, and mediastinum shifted to the right

HEMORRHAGE

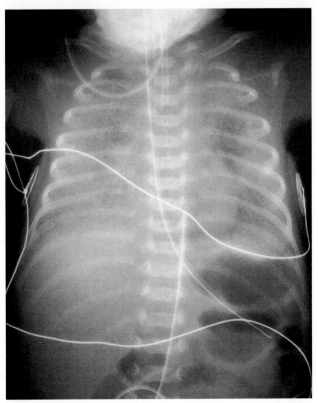

FIGURE 4–42. Pulmonary hemorrhage

AIR BLOCK SYNDROMES

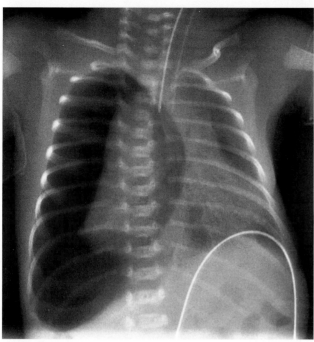

Pneumothorax

FIGURE 4–43. Right pneumothorax, compliant lung collapsed

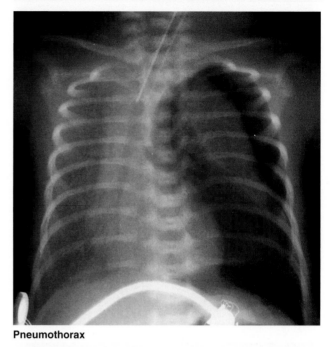

Pneumothorax

FIGURE 4–45. Left pneumothorax, lung poorly compliant

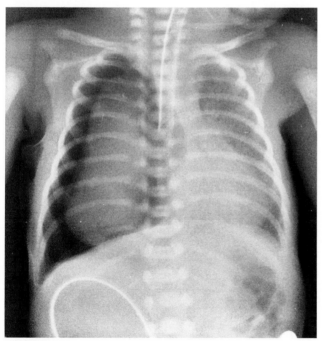

Pneumothorax

FIGURE 4–44. Right pneumothorax, lung poorly compliant

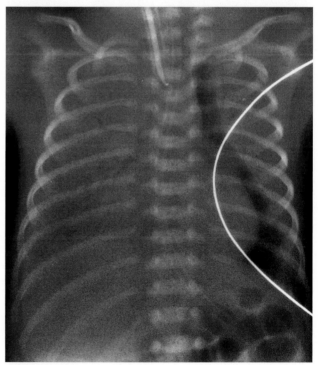

Pneumothorax

FIGURE 4–46. Left paramediastinal pneumothorax

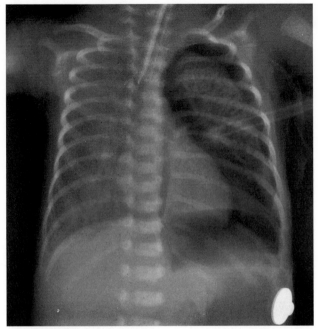

Pneumothorax

FIGURE 4–47. Left subpulmonic pneumothorax

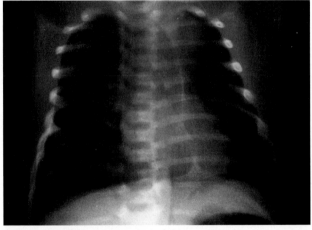

Pneumothorax

FIGURE 4–48. Anterior mediastinal line defined by bilateral pneumothoraces

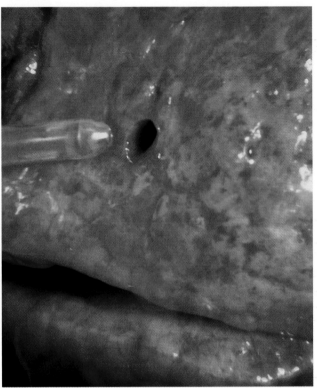

Pneumothorax

FIGURE 4–49. Punctured lung from a chest tube

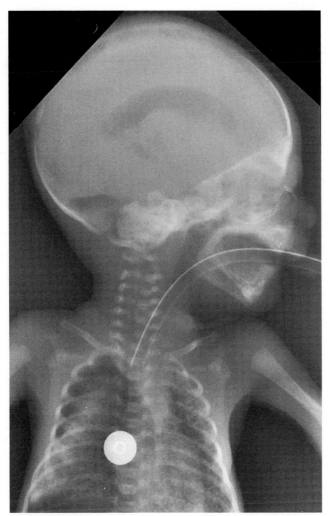

Pneumothorax

FIGURE 4–50. Right tension pneumothorax and pneumoencephalo-gram

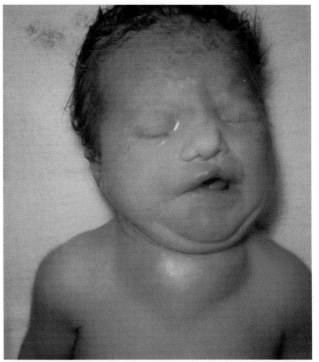

Pneumomediastinum

FIGURE 4–51. Neck distention with air

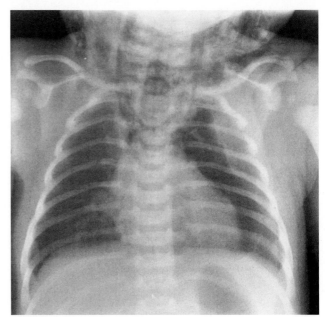

Pneumomediastinum

FIGURE 4–52. Air in the neck seen radiographically

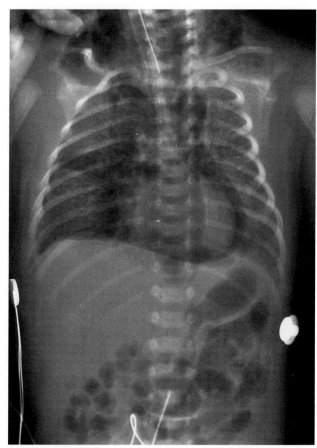

Pneumomediastinum

FIGURE 4–53. Large pneumomediastinum surrounding the heart and dissecting into the neck

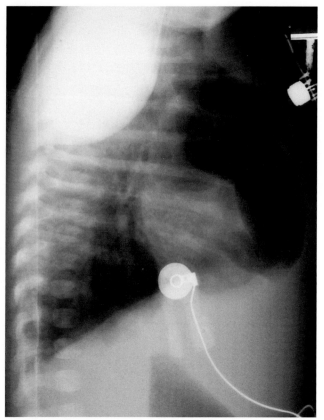

Pneumomediastinum

FIGURE 4–55. Lateral radiograph: upper mediastinal air

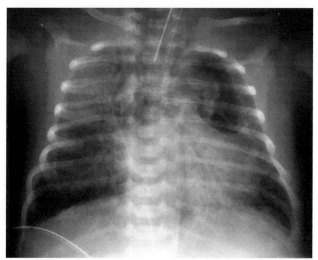

Pneumomediastinum

FIGURE 4–54. Anteroposterior radiograph: air in upper mediastinum

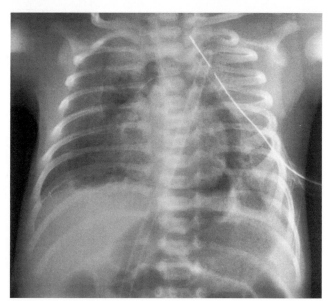

Pneumomediastinum

FIGURE 4–56. Sail sign—thymic elevation

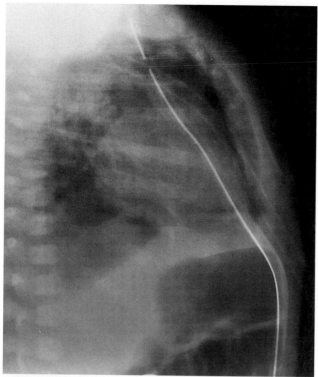

Pneumomediastinum

FIGURE 4–57. Lateral—elevation of the thymus

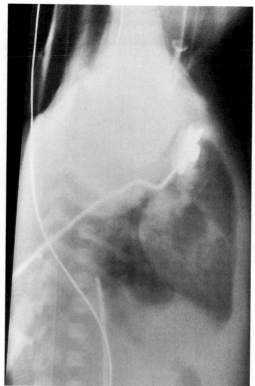

Pneumomediastinum

FIGURE 4–59. Lateral—cardiac compression

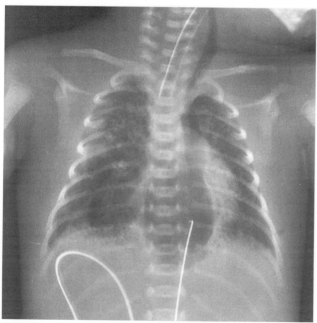

Pneumomediastinum

FIGURE 4–58. Air anterior to the heart

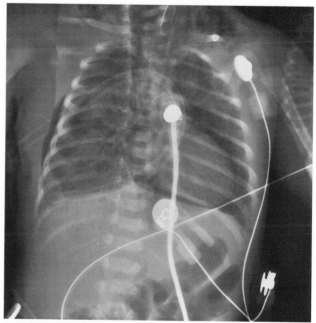

Pneumomediastinum

FIGURE 4–60. Pneumomediastinum and left pneumothorax

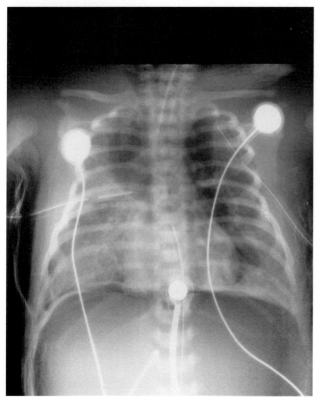

Pneumomediastinum

FIGURE 4–61. Pneumoperitoneum dissected from a pneumomediastinum

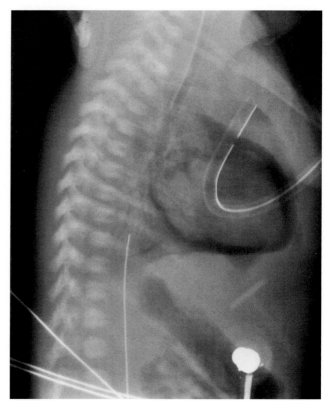

Pneumopericardium

FIGURE 4–63. Lateral: air confined to pericardium

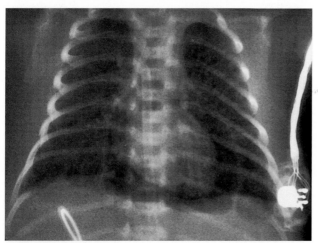

Pneumopericardium

FIGURE 4–62. Anteroposterior film: pericardium distinct

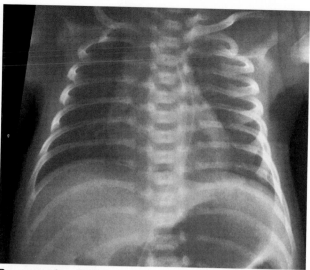

Pneumopericardium

FIGURE 4–65. Decompression with pericardial catheter

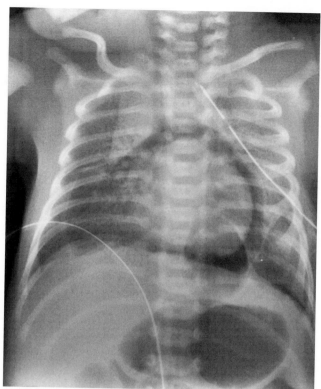

Pneumopericardium

FIGURE 4–64. Anteroposterior view: distended pericardial sac

AIR BLOCK SEQUENCE IN A PRETERM BABY

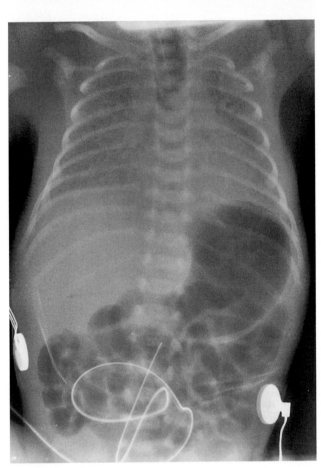

FIGURE 4–66. Early surfactant deficiency

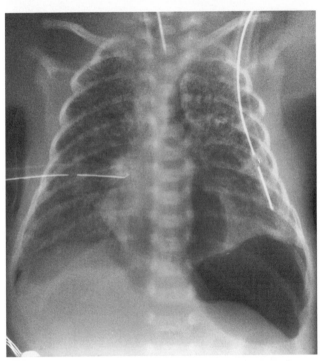

FIGURE 4–68. Left pneumothorax under tension, depressed left diaphragm

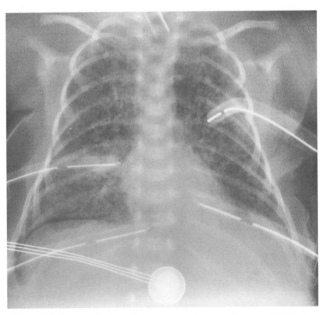

FIGURE 4–69. Resolution of the pneumothorax after an additional chest tube insertion

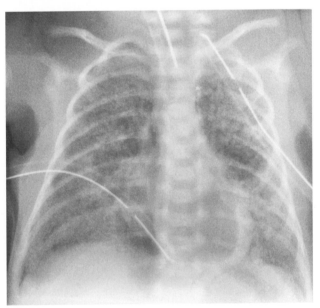

FIGURE 4–67. Pneumomediastinum, bilateral chest tubes

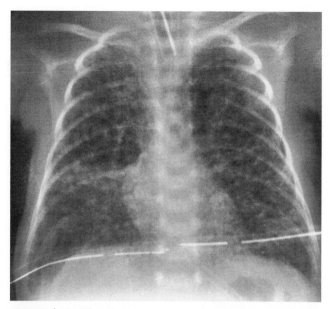

FIGURE 4–70. Bilateral air trapping with right middle lobe atelectasis

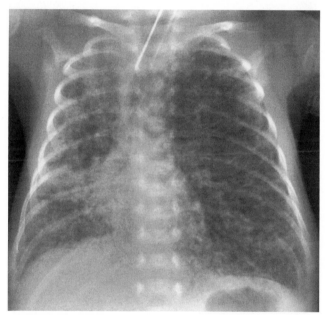

FIGURE 4–71. Interstitial emphysema of left lung, increased right middle lobe atelectasis

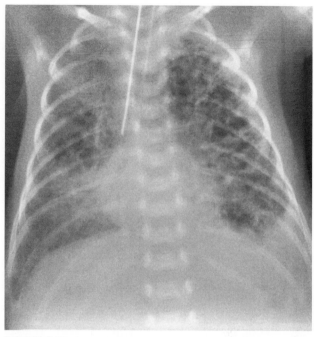

FIGURE 4–72. Intentional right main stem intubation to collapse the left lung

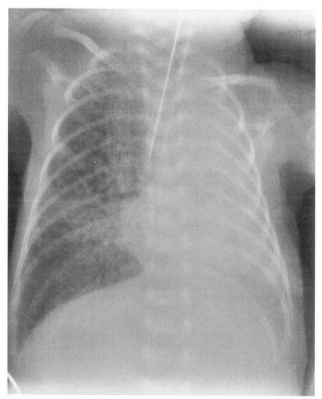

FIGURE 4–73. Atelectasis of entire left lung

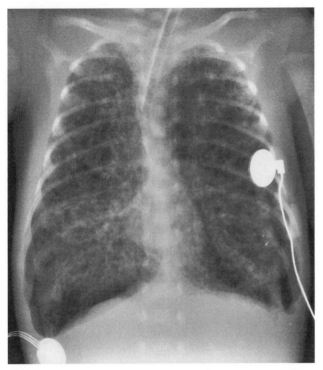

FIGURE 4–74. Severe gas trapping—depressed diaphragm, small mediastinum

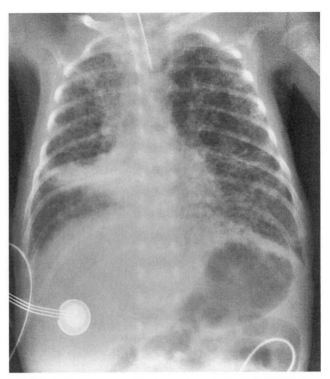

FIGURE 4–76. Improved with plate atelectasis of right middle lobe

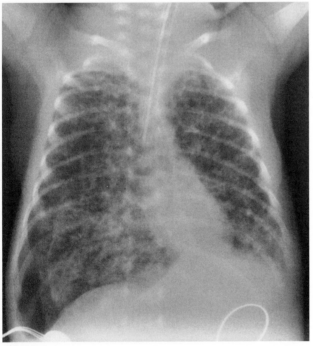

FIGURE 4–75. Asymmetric hyperexpansion of right lung with small pneumothorax

"NO CARDIA"—SOME CONDITIONS RESULT IN THE RELATIVE ABSENCE OF THE CARDIAC SILHOUETTE RADIOGRAPHICALLY

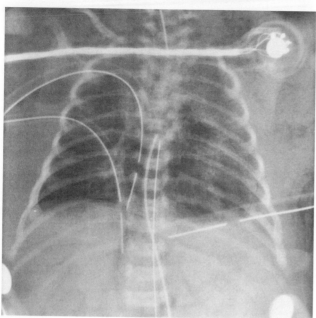

Intracardiac Air from a Ruptured Bronchus

FIGURE 4–77. Anteroposterior film of air-filled heart

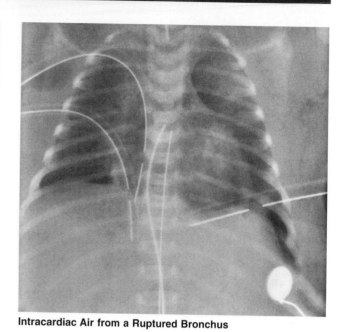

Intracardiac Air from a Ruptured Bronchus

FIGURE 4–79. Anteroposterior view after volume replacement

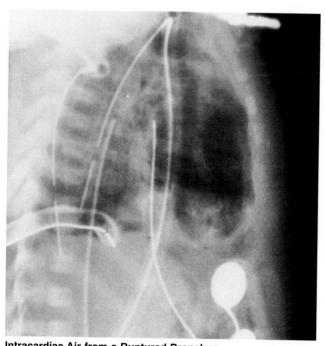

Intracardiac Air from a Ruptured Bronchus

FIGURE 4–78. Lateral film demonstrating cardiac septum

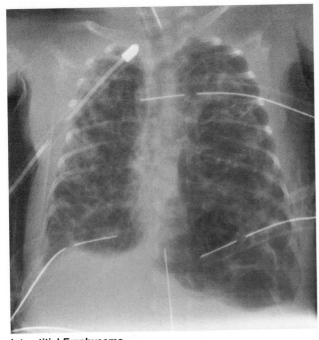

Interstitial Emphysema

FIGURE 4–80. Severe interstitial emphysema

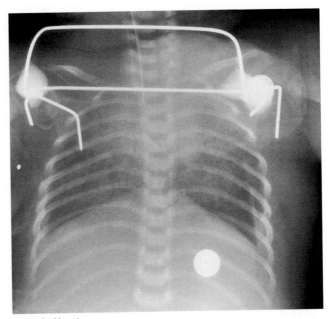

Ectopic Heart

FIGURE 4–81. Ectopic heart

PULMONARY CYSTS

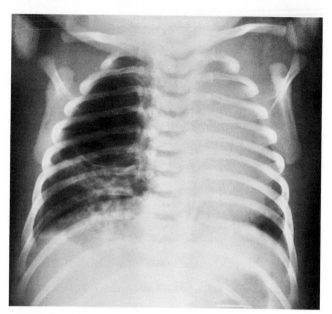

FIGURE 4–82. Hyperlucent right lung

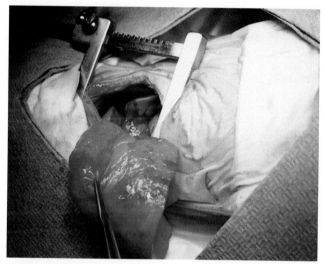

FIGURE 4–83. Surgical specimen of cystic right middle and lower lobes

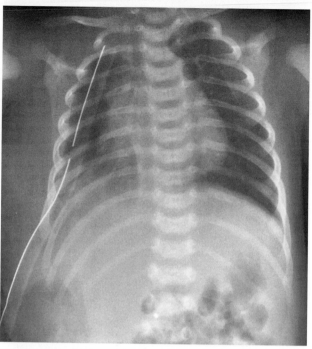

FIGURE 4–84. Postoperative chest radiograph: normal left lung

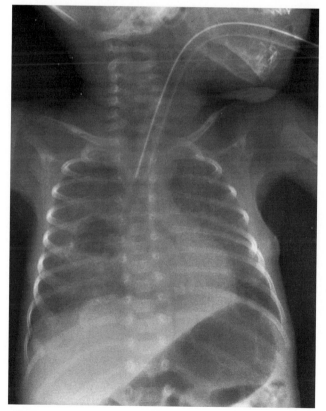

FIGURE 4–85. Right perihilar cyst

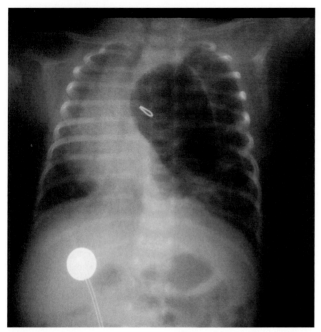

FIGURE 4-86. Acquired left pulmonary cyst, mediastinal shift, and depressed diaphragm

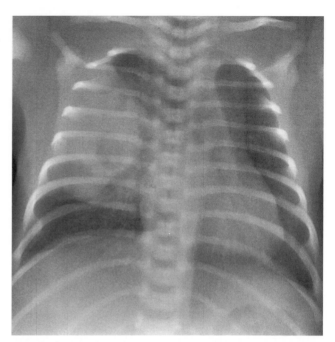

FIGURE 4-88. Cystic adenomatous malformation of right lung

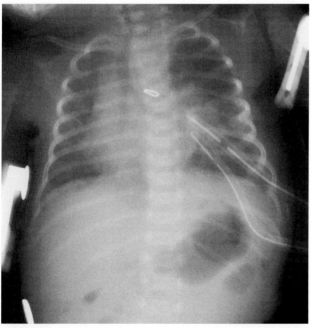

FIGURE 4-87. Postoperative chest radiograph with well-expanded left upper lobe

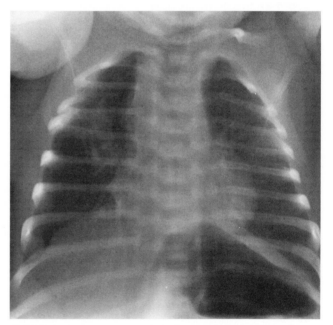

FIGURE 4-89. Postoperative relatively normal chest radiograph

CHYLOTHORAX

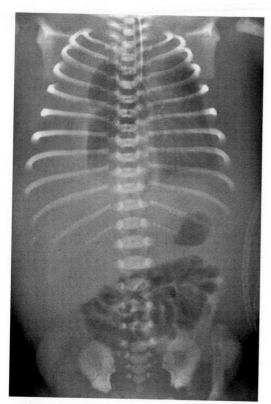

FIGURE 4–90. Radiograph: large right chylothorax

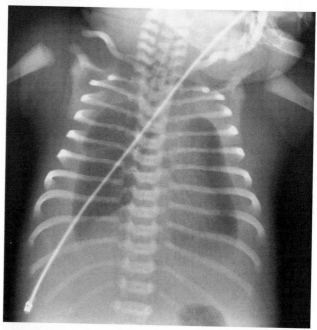

FIGURE 4–92. Bilateral chylothoraces

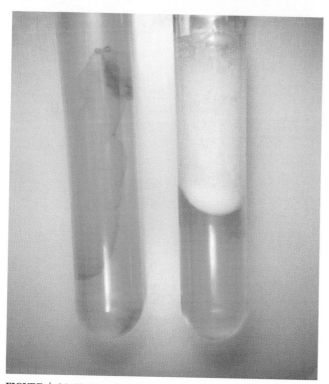

FIGURE 4–91. Fluid aspirated—serous, with numerous lymphocytes and protein

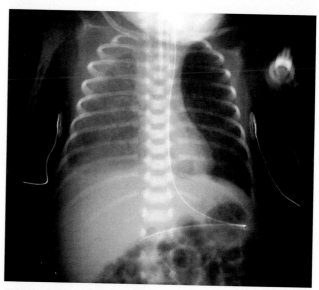

FIGURE 4–93. Pleural effusion

CONGENITAL DIAPHRAGMATIC HERNIA

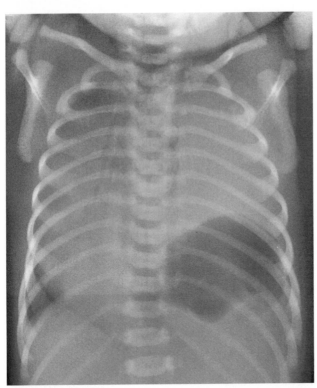

Left Foramen of Bochdalek Hernia

FIGURE 4–94. Stomach in left chest, dense left hemithorax

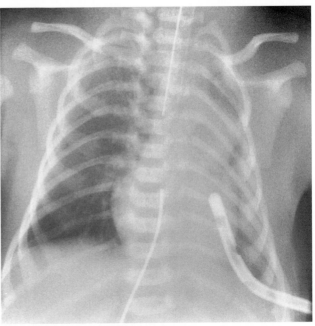

Left Foramen of Bochdalek Hernia

FIGURE 4–96. Postoperative radiograph: normal right lung expansion and limited left lung aeration

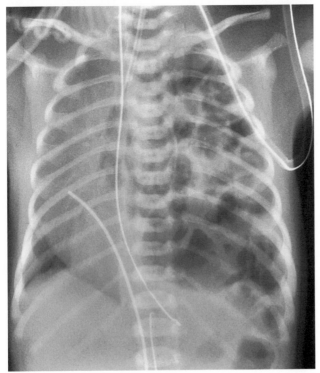

Left Foramen of Bochdalek Hernia

FIGURE 4–95. Air-filled small intestine in left hemithorax

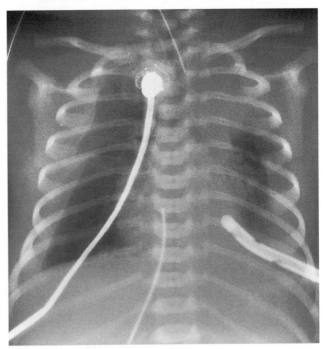

Left Foramen of Bochdalek Hernia

FIGURE 4–97. Bilateral pleural effusions several days later

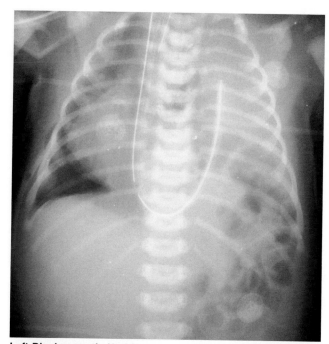

Left Diaphragmatic Hernia

FIGURE 4–98. Nasogastric tube tip in left chest

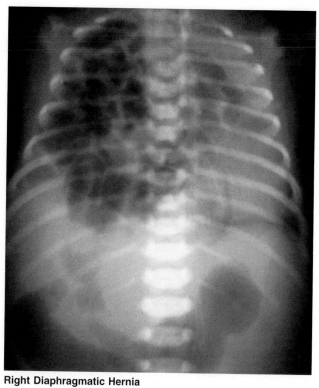

Right Diaphragmatic Hernia

FIGURE 4–100. Gas-filled intestine in right hemithorax

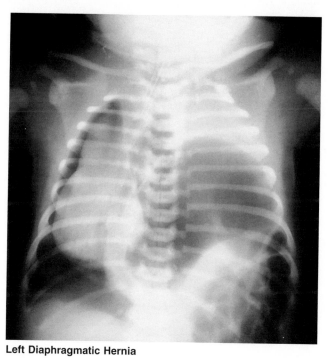

Left Diaphragmatic Hernia

FIGURE 4–99. Air-filled stomach in left chest

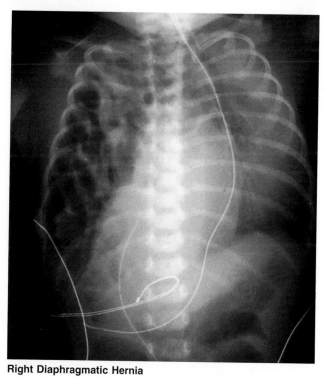

Right Diaphragmatic Hernia

FIGURE 4–101. Bowel and liver in right chest

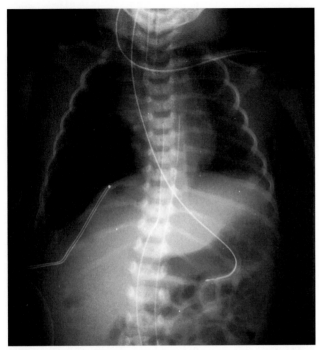

Right Diaphragmatic Hernia

FIGURE 4–102. Postoperative radiograph with taut, repaired diaphragm

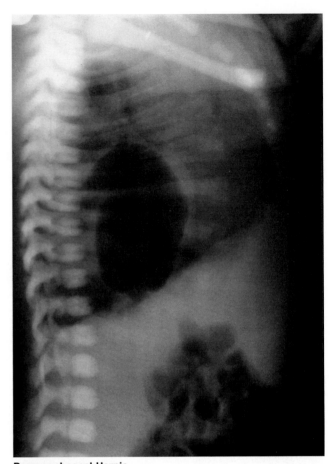

Paraesophageal Hernia

FIGURE 4–104. Lateral: gas-filled intestine in posterior chest

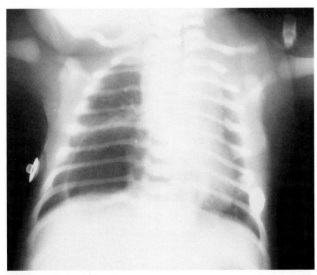

Paraesophageal Hernia

FIGURE 4–103. Air-filled pouch in right chest

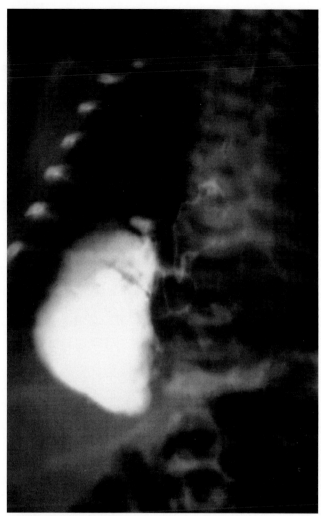

Paraesophageal Hernia

FIGURE 4–105. Contrast material defining the pouch

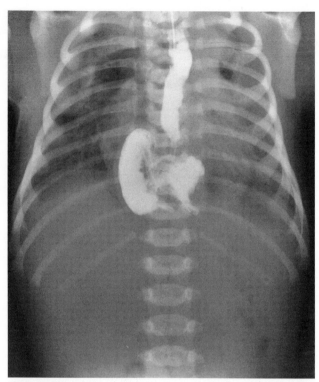

Morgagni Hernia

FIGURE 106. Morgagni hernia demonstrated by barium swallow

DIAPHRAGM DYSFUNCTION

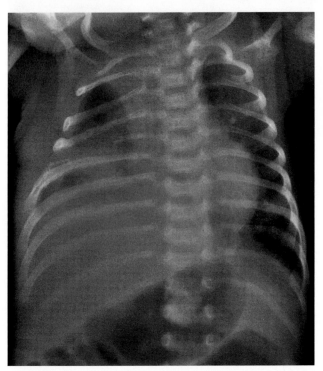

FIGURE 4–107. Paralyzed right diaphragm postoperatively

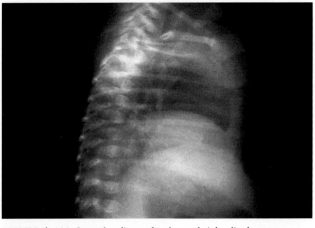

FIGURE 4–109. Lateral radiograph: elevated right diaphragm

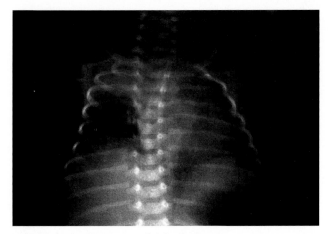

FIGURE 4–108. Eventration of right diaphragm

SELECTED REFERENCES

Jones KL. (1997) Smith's Recognizable Patterns of Human Malformation. Philadelphia, WB Saunders.

Poling RA and Fox WW. (1998) Fetal and Neonatal Physiology. Philadelphia, WB Saunders, Chapters 78-94.

Respiratory Medicine (June 1994) Pediatr Clin North Am 41(3).

Taeusch HW and Ballard R. (1998) Avery's Diseases of the Newborn. Philadelphia, WB Saunders, Chapters 48-60.-

Cardiology

Congenital abnormalities of the cardiovascular system present as a wide variety of clinical signs and symptoms. Children can have any variation from catastrophic emergencies in the first minutes of life to insignificant abnormalities that never cause a problem. The abnormalities pictured in this section attempt to give a glimpse of the breadth but certainly not a statistical representation of the types of abnormalities found.

Although the abnormalities described have a broad array of etiologies, the majority are malformations; disruptions or deformations are much less common.

The frequency of these abnormalities is often quoted at approximately 8 of every 1000 live births, which amount to 10% of all congenital malformations. It's important to remember that many of these will not be symptomatic or found in the newborn period.

A brief outline of the embryology of cardiac development is often helpful in understanding the etiology and timing of problems (Table 5-1). In the second week of gestation, mesodermal cells migrate in a usually orderly fashion to form a tube that fuses in a cranial to caudad

fashion. During the third week, the tube is complete and the heart begins to beat. As the tube continues to elongate, it bends and lines up the great vessels with the atrium and future ventricles. At approximately 36 days the ventricular septum and the septum between the pulmonary artery and the aorta are formed. Also in the busy fifth week valves are formed from endocardial tissue, and the ostium primum closes. Epicardial cells then migrate to form initially the cardiac veins and capillaries, which then push their way up to the aorta and ultimately become the coronary arteries. By the end of the sixth week the membranous ventricular septum is formed, and, it is hoped, an anatomically correct heart beats vigorously in this still very tiny fetus.

In the majority of children who have congenital heart disease, there is no obvious etiology. An increased frequency of cardiac anomalies is found in children with genetic abnormalities (Table 5-2). Trisomy 21, 18, and 13 all have a markedly increased risk of cardiac abnormalities. Furthermore, there are a number of single gene defects such as Holt-Oram (autosomal dominant abnor-

TABLE 5-1

CARDIOVASCULAR SYSTEM DEVELOPMENT		
GESTATIONAL AGE	DEVELOPMENT PROCESS	CONGENITAL ABNORMALITY
21–28 days	Pericardium forms	—
30 days	Heart tube loops to the right	Situs inversus
30 days	Proximal pulmonary vein	Anomalous pulmonary veins
38 days	Formation of muscular ventricular septum	Ventricular septal defect or single ventricle
38 days	Septation of pulmonary artery and aorta	Truncus arteriosus
38–40 days	Resorption of tissue between aorta and left ventricle	Aortic valve atresia or stenosis
40 days	Endocardial tissue; ostium primum closes	Tricuspid valve defects; ostium primum atrial septal defect
44 days	Membranous ventricular septum closes	Membranous ventricular septal defect
7.5 wks	Pulmonary vein fuses into left atrium	Anomalous pulmonary venous return
8 wks	Atrioventricular bundle	
	Sinus venosus absorbed into right auricle	—
9–12 wks	Bronchial arteries	
38–40 wks	Rapid decrease in pulmonary vascular resistance (10-15 hrs after birth)	Patent ductus arteriosus
		Persistent pulmonary hypertension
	Closure of foramen ovale, ductus arteriosus, and ductus venosus	

TABLE 5-2

CONGENITAL HEART DISEASE ASSOCIATED WITH COMMON CHROMOSOMAL ABNORMALITIES

GROUP	INCIDENCE (%)	DEFECT IN ORDER OF FREQUENCY
General population	1	VSD
		PDA
Trisomy 21	40	Endocardial cushion defect
		VSD
		PDA
		ASD
		Aberrant subclavian artery
Trisomy 18	90	VSD
		PDA
		ASD
Trisomy 13	80	VSD
		PDA
		ASD
		Dextroposition
4p minus	40	ASD
		VSD
5p minus	20	VSD
(cri du chat syndrome)		PDA
XO (Turner syndrome)	30	Aortic coarctation
		Aortic stenosis

ASD, atrial septal defect; PDA, patent ductus arteriosus; VSD, ventricular septal defect.

mality with atrial septal defects) and Laurence-Moon-Biedl (autosomal recessive, ventricular septal defects). Uncommonly, cardiac defects are caused by environmental factors. The use of prescription drugs such as warfarin, diphenylhydantoin, or antimetabolites has been reported to increase the incidence of cardiac malformations. Infections, such as rubella causing peripheral pulmonary stenosis, or connective tissue diseases, such as maternal systemic lupus erythematosus causing electrical conduction problems, are rare.

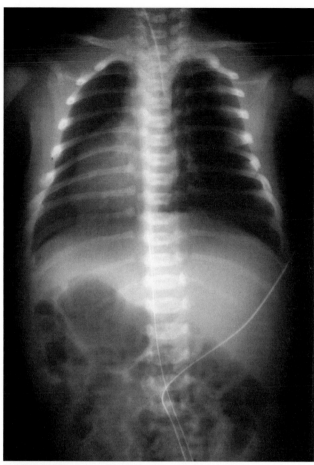

Dextrocardia

FIGURE 5–1. Dextrocardia with situs inversus

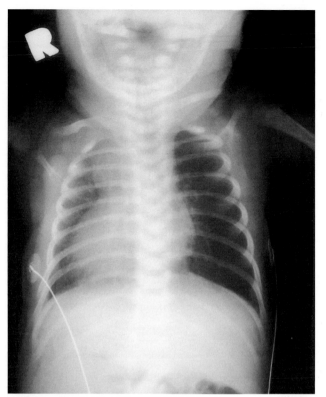

Dextrocardia

FIGURE 5–2. Dextrocardia with situs solitus

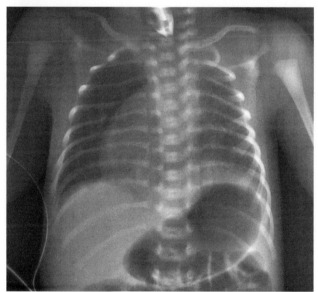

Dextrocardia

FIGURE 5–3. Dextrocardia with tracheoesophageal fistula

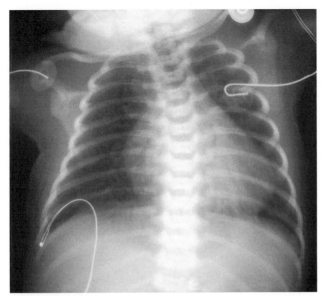

FIGURE 5–4. DiGeorge syndrome: aortic stenosis with absent thymus

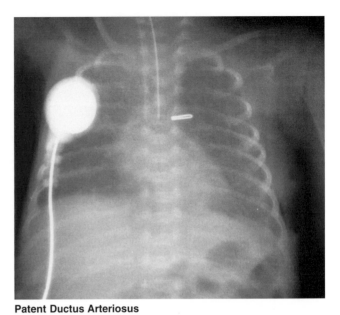

Patent Ductus Arteriosus

FIGURE 5–6. Decreased heart size and clearer lung fields following PDA ligation

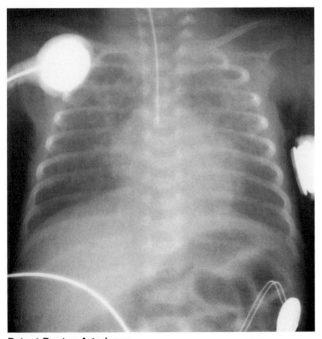

Patent Ductus Arteriosus

FIGURE 5–5. Congestive heart failure with enlarged heart due to left to right shunt

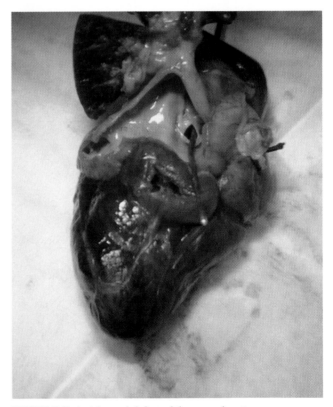

FIGURE 5–7. Atrial septal defect of the secundum type

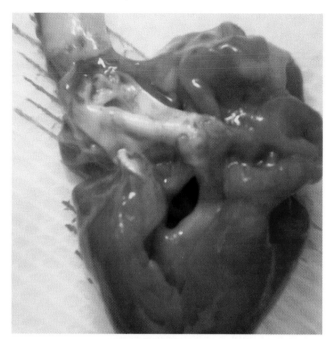

FIGURE 5–8. Ventricular septal defect

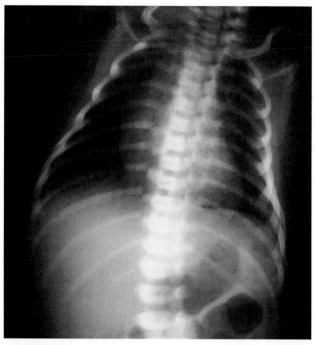

FIGURE 5–10. Truncus arteriosus with poor pulmonary blood flow

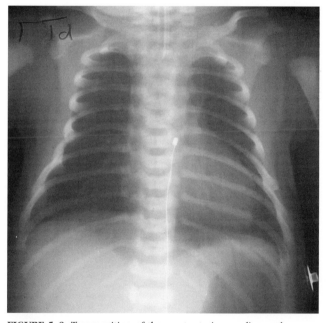

FIGURE 5–9. Transposition of the great arteries, cardiomegaly, narrow superior mediastinum

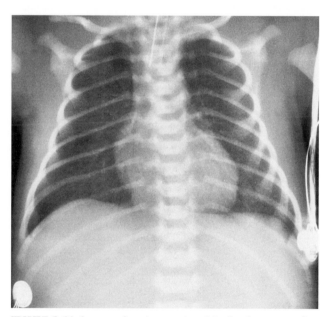

FIGURE 5–11. Severe pulmonic stenosis, minimal pulmonary perfusion

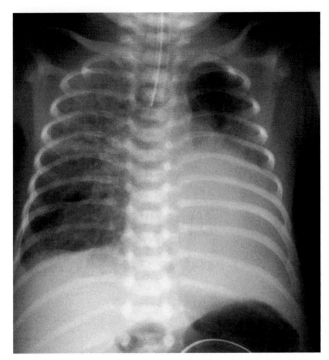

FIGURE 5–12. Tetralogy of Fallot, cardiomegaly

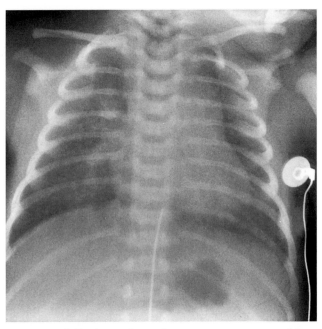

FIGURE 5–14. Total anomalous pulmonary venous return, perihilar venous congestion

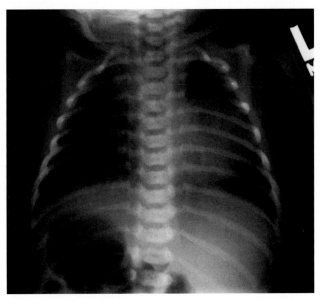

FIGURE 5–13. Tricuspid atresia, pulmonary perfusion via patent ductus arteriosus

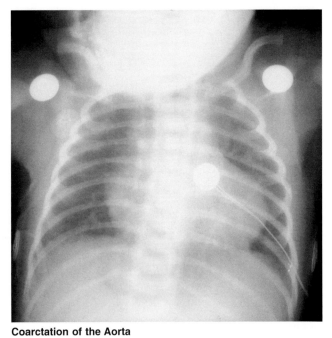

Coarctation of the Aorta

FIGURE 5–15. Cardiomegaly

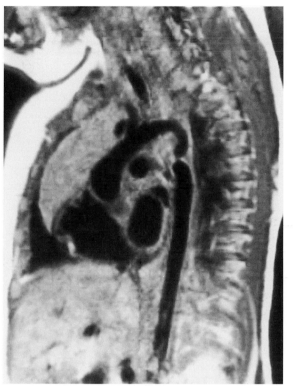

Coarctation of the Aorta

FIGURE 5–16. MRI demonstrating a coarctation of the descending aorta

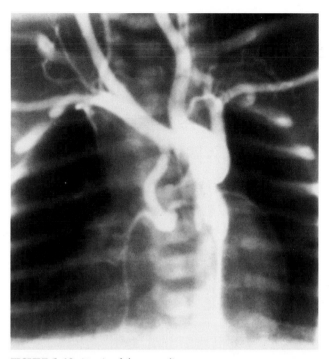

FIGURE 5–18. Atresia of the ascending aorta

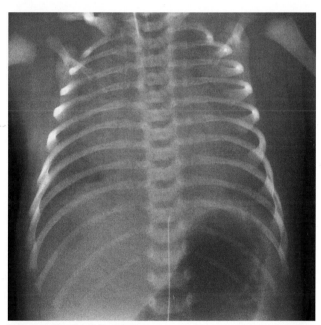

Hypoplastic Heart Syndrome

FIGURE 5–19. Congestive heart failure with cardiomegaly, hypoplastic left heart

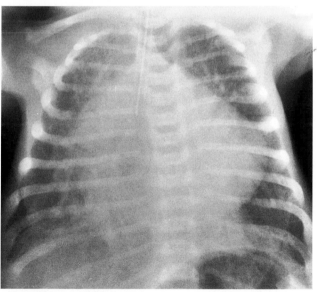

Coarctation of the Aorta

FIGURE 5–17. Severe cardiomegaly due to aortic coarctation with ventricular septal defect

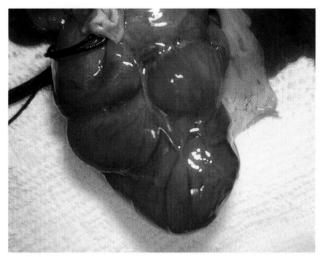

Hypoplastic Heart Syndrome

FIGURE 5–20. Postmortem heart with a small left ventricle

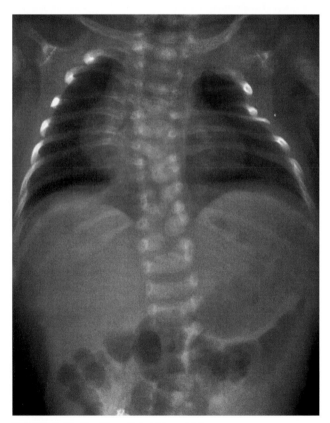

FIGURE 5–21. Double outlet right ventricle

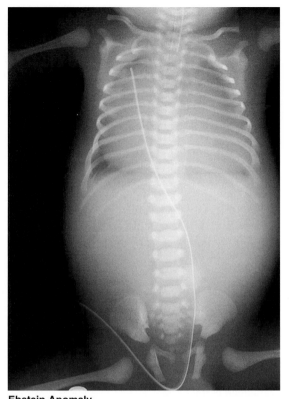

Ebstein Anomaly

FIGURE 5–22. Massive cardiomegaly

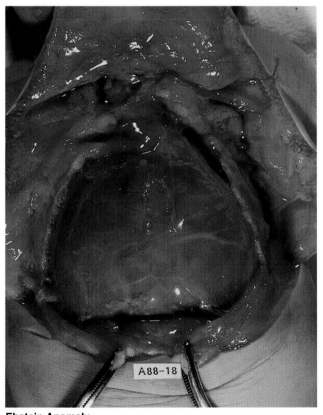

Ebstein Anomaly

FIGURE 5–23. Postmortem grossly enlarged heart

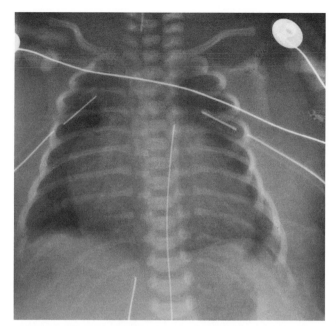

FIGURE 5–24. Hydrops and cardiomegaly due to fetal supraventricular tachycardia

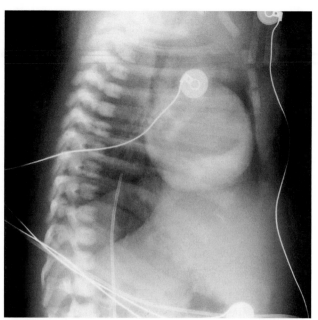

Cardiac Catheterization: Contrast in the Pericardium Due to Atrial Perforation

FIGURE 5–26. Lateral view of radiodense pericardial sac

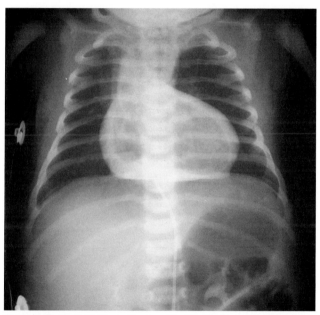

Cardiac Catheterization: Contrast in the Pericardium Due to Atrial Perforation

FIGURE 5–25. Anteroposterior view of radiodense pericardial sac

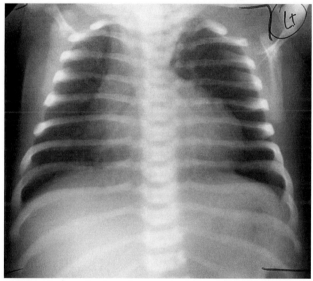

Cardiac Catheterization: Contrast in the Pericardium Due to Atrial Perforation

FIGURE 5–27. Clearance of contrast

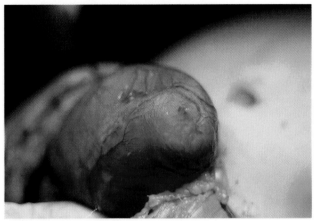

Myocardial Infarction

FIGURE 5–28. Gross specimen: pale apex of the ventricle

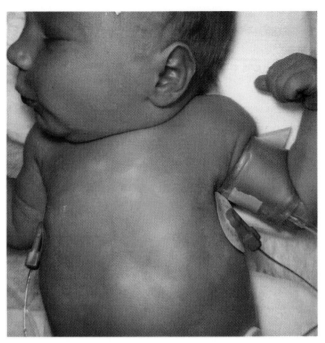

FIGURE 5–30. Cutaneous flush due to prostaglandin E_1 administration to maintain pulmonary flow via the ductus

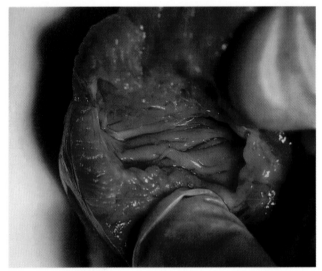

Myocardial Infarction

FIGURE 5–29. Cross-section: thinned ventricle at apex

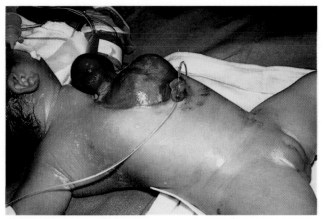

Ectopic Heart

FIGURE 5–31. External structures of the heart and mediastinum

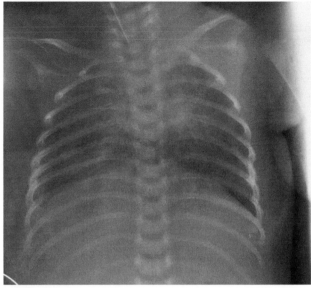

Ectopic Heart

FIGURE 5–32. Radiograph revealing small thorax and decreased lung volume

SELECTED REFERENCES

Jones KL. (1997) Smith's Recognizable Patterns of Human Malformation. Philadelphia, WB Saunders.

Long WA. (1990) Fetal and Neonatal Cardiology. Philadelphia, WB Saunders.

Lott JW. Assessment and management of cardiovascular dysfunction. *In* Kenner C, Brueggemeyer A, and Gunderson LP, Eds. (1993) Comprehensive Neonatal Nursing. Philadelphia, WB Saunders, pp 335–391.

Polin RA and Fox WW. (1998) Fetal and Neonatal Physiology. Philadelphia, WB Saunders, Chapters 78–94.

Taeusch HW and Ballard RA. (1998) Avery's Diseases of the Newborn. Philadelphia, WB Saunders, Chapters 61–65.

6 Neurology

Abnormalities of the central nervous system (CNS) vary from the obvious and devastating anencephaly to very subtle and clinically insignificant minor variations in nervous system structure. The development of the central nervous system is outlined in Table 6-1.

The etiology for these abnormalities is often unclear and multifactorial. Certainly there are genetic connections with the CNS abnormalities seen commonly in children afflicted with trisomy 13 or trisomy 18. The increased frequency of myelomeningocele in certain ethnic groups or siblings of affected individuals implies a genetic link. This group of anomalies seems to show a definite correlation between prenatal folate intake and the incidence of neural tube defects. Infections at critical times of fetal development have been associated with both aqueductal stenosis and agenesis of the corpus callosum. A wide variety of in utero insults, including metabolic defects, vitamin deficiencies, and alcohol exposure, have been associated with abnormalities of cell migration or proliferation.

The incidence of these varies markedly through different populations, often related to ethnicity, socioeconomic status, and geographic location (Table 6-2). Some abnormalities such as hydrocephalus have been noted to be more common than 1 in 1000, whereas others are very rare or have no clear incidence. In evaluating incidence, it is important to note that many abnormalities (e.g., agenesis of the corpus callosum) have a very high incidence of associated anomalies in other organ systems.

TABLE 6-1

CNS DEVELOPMENT AND ABNORMALITIES		
TIMING	CNS DEVELOPMENTAL EVENT	COMPLICATIONS
16-24 days	Failure of anterior neural tube closure	Anencephaly
<26 days	Failure of caudal neural tube closure	Myelomeningocele
by 6th wk	Cleavage of the cerebral vesicle	Holoprosencephaly
by 8th wk	Failure of neuronal proliferation	Micrencephaly
5-12 wks	Abnormal formation of the cerebellar vermis and roof of 4th ventricle	Dandy-Walker malformation
9-20 wks	Failure of appropriate development of internal cerebral crossing fibers	Agenesis of the corpus callosum
12-20 wks	Failure of appropriate cellular migration	Schizencephaly, lissencephaly, etc.
15-17 wks	Failure of appropriate patency of the aqueduct	Aqueductal stenosis

TABLE 6–2

INCIDENCE AND ETIOLOGY OF CNS MALFORMATIONS

ABNORMALITY	SUSPECTED ETIOLOGY	INCIDENCE
Anencephaly	Genetic + environmental	0.5–2/1000 (US)
Myelomeningocele	Genetic (ethnic, siblings), environmental (especially dietary folate)	0.2–0.4/100,000 live births
Holoprosencephaly	Genetic, especially trisomy 13, trisomy 18, autosomal dominant and recessive	1 in 15,000 live births
Micrencephaly	Variable genetic and teratogenic suggested etiologies, including alcohol, cytomegalovirus, etc.	Not known
Dandy-Walker cysts	Increased incidence in siblings suggests genetic link	1 in 3000/1 in 10,000
Agenesis of the corpus callosum	Often unclear, suspected metabolic disease, vitamin deficiency, alcohol-related	Not known (very rare, often an isolated finding)
Schizencephaly, lissencephaly	Genetic (Miller-Dieker syndrome), infectious, hereditary, metabolic abnormalities have all been implicated	Extremely variable
Aqueduct of Sylvius stenosis	Infectious agents suspected, X link reported	Approximately 1/3 of all hydrocephalus (0.1–3.5/1000)

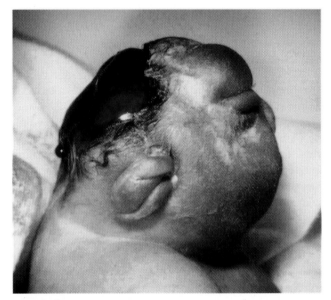

FIGURE 6–1. Anencephaly, lateral view

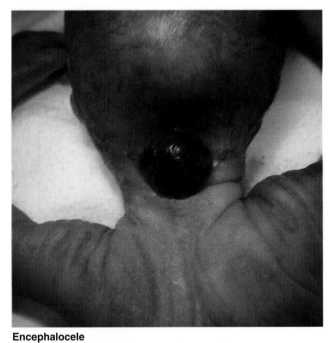

Encephalocele

FIGURE 6–3. Posterior at the base of the skull

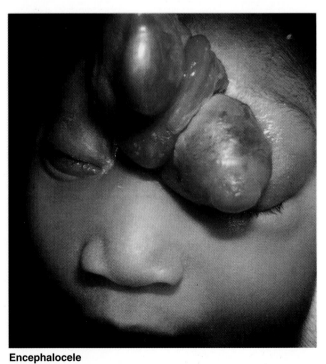

Encephalocele

FIGURE 6–2. Anterior view

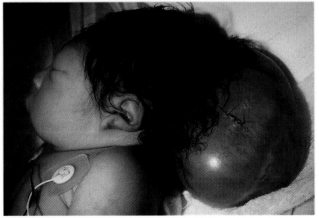

Encephalocele

FIGURE 6–4. Large posterior encephalocele

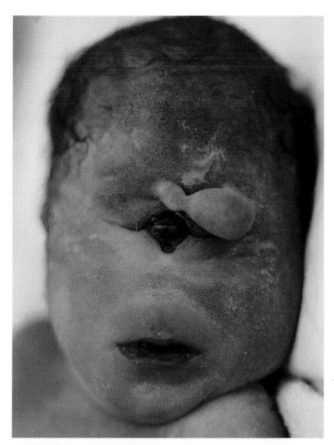

FIGURE 6–5. Holoprosencephaly

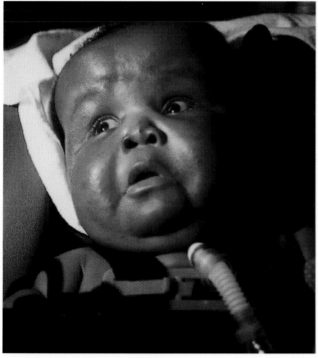

FIGURE 6–6. Macrocephaly, familial

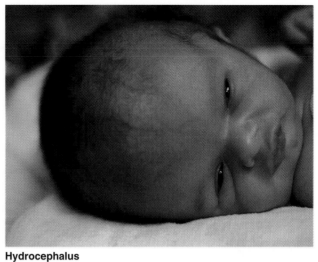

Hydrocephalus

FIGURE 6–7. X linked—stenosis of the aqueduct of Sylvius

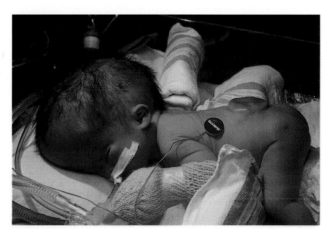

Hydrocephalus

FIGURE 6–8. Hydranencephaly with cerebral dysgenesis

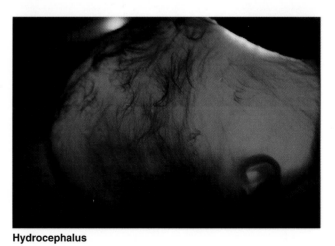

Hydrocephalus

FIGURE 6–9. Transillumination

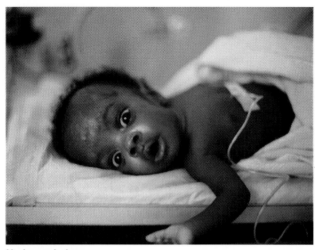

Hydrocephalus

FIGURE 6–10. Sunset sign

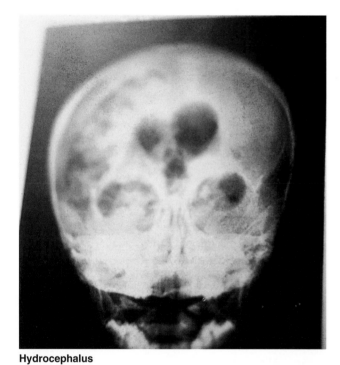

Hydrocephalus

FIGURE 6–11. Pneumoencephalogram demonstrating hydrocephalus (1960)

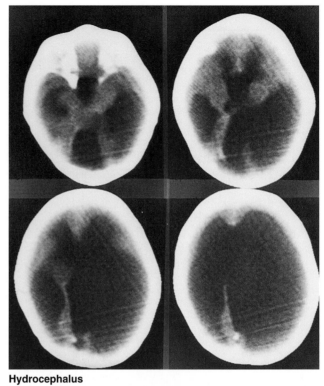

Hydrocephalus

FIGURE 6–12. CT scan: four views of severe hydrocephalus

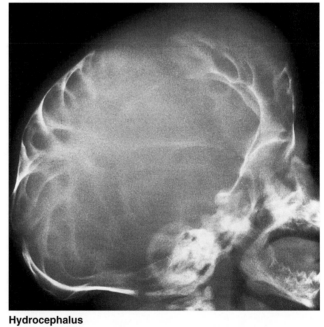

Hydrocephalus

FIGURE 6–13. Thinned skull (Lukenshädel) from increased intracranial pressure

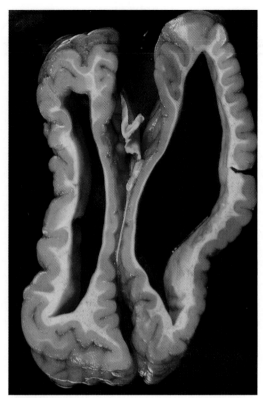

Hydrocephalus

FIGURE 6–14. Thinned cerebral cortex with grossly enlarged ventricles

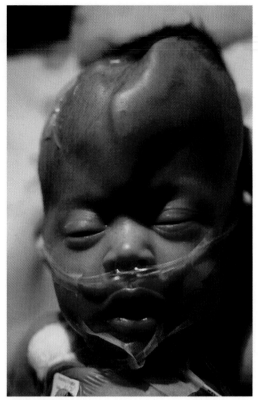

Hydrocephalus

FIGURE 6–16. Overlapped sutures following ventriculoperitoneal shunt and decompression

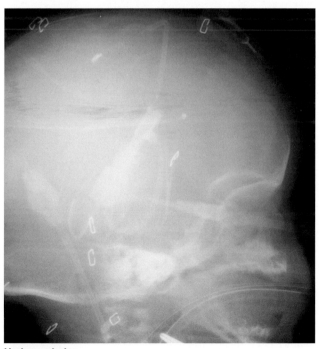

Hydrocephalus

FIGURE 6–15. Ventriculoperitoneal shunt

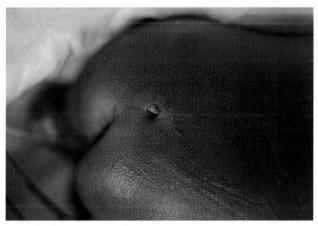

FIGURE 6–17. Sacral dimple

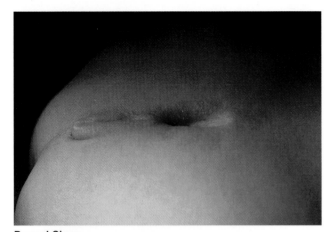

Dermal Sinus

FIGURE 6–18. External view

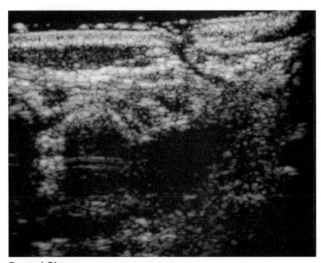

Dermal Sinus

FIGURE 6–19. MRI demonstrating sinus tract

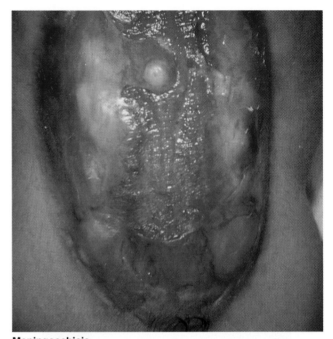

Meningoschisis

FIGURE 6–20. Thoracolumbar meningoschisis

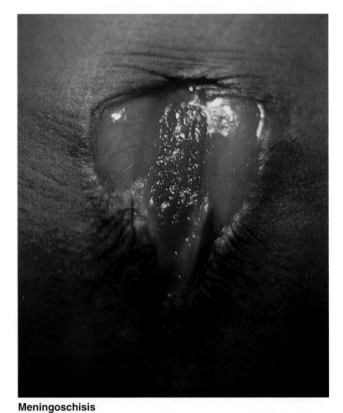

Meningoschisis

FIGURE 6–21. Lumbar meningoschisis with hair

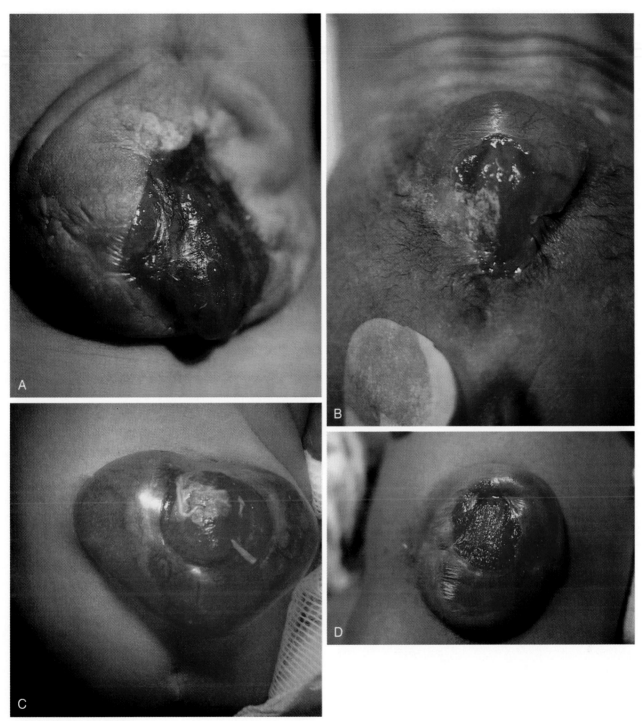

Meningomyelocele Series

FIGURE 6–22. A-D, Variations of size, shape, and membranes covering neural elements

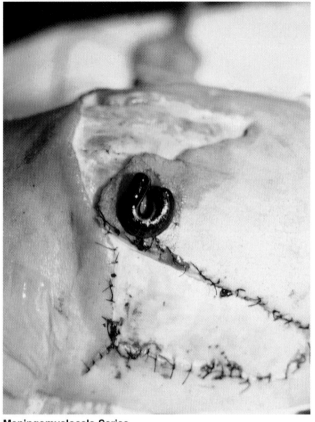

Meningomyelocele Series

FIGURE 6–23. Leeches used to maintain blood flow to the cutaneous flap following the repair of a large meningomyelocele

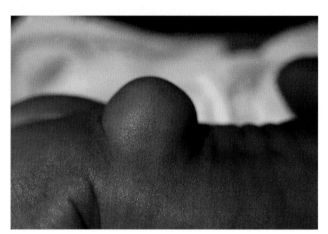

FIGURE 6–24. Lipomeningocele

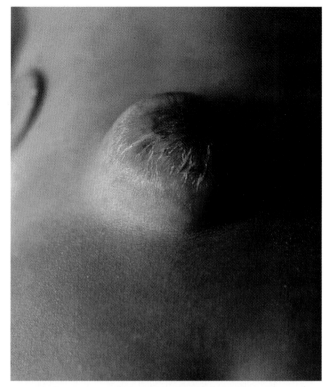

FIGURE 6–25. Hemangiomeningocele

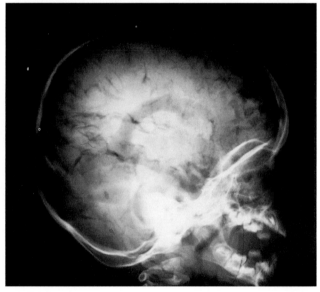

FIGURE 6–26. Pneumoencephalogram demonstrating cortical aplasia

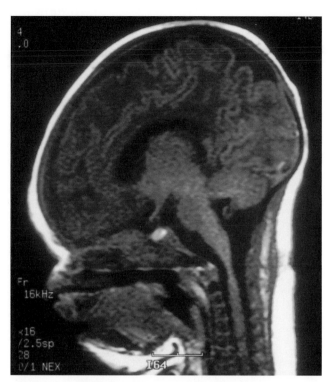

FIGURE 6–27. MRI of cerebellar dysgenesis

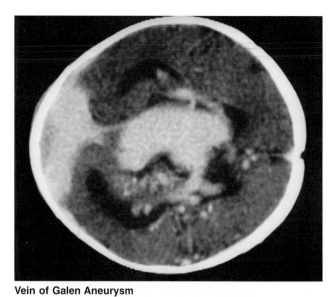

Vein of Galen Aneurysm

FIGURE 6–29. CT scan showing vascular enlargement

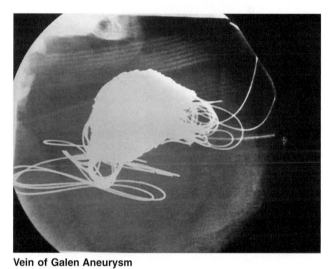

Vein of Galen Aneurysm

FIGURE 6–30. Coils inserted to ablate the aneurysm

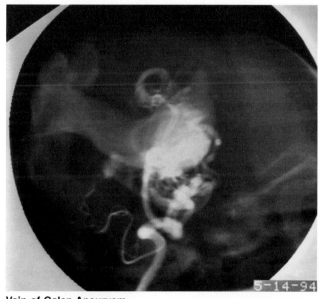

Vein of Galen Aneurysm

FIGURE 6–28. Venogram

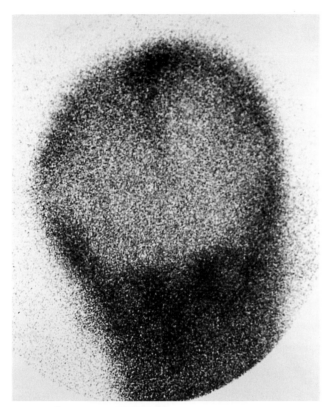

FIGURE 6–31. Brain scan with no flow—postasphyxia

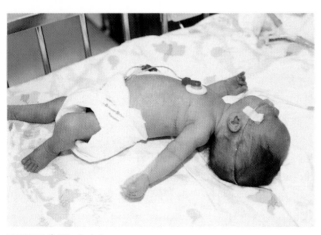

FIGURE 6–32. Opisthotonos

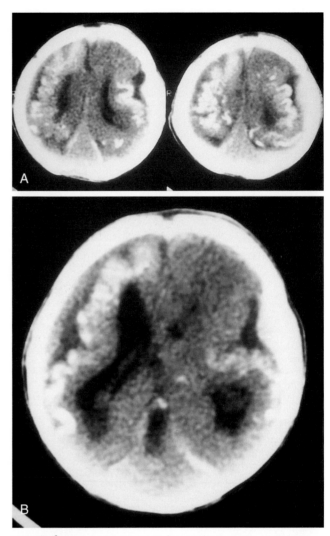

FIGURE 6–33. A and B, Sturge-Weber syndrome—two cross-sectional MRI views at different levels showing vascular involvement of the cerebral cortex

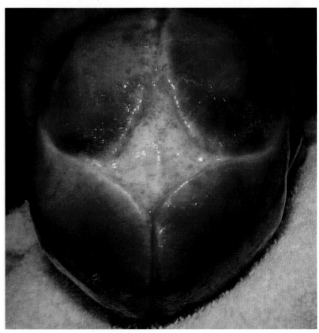

FIGURE 6–34. Anterior fontanelle—postmortem

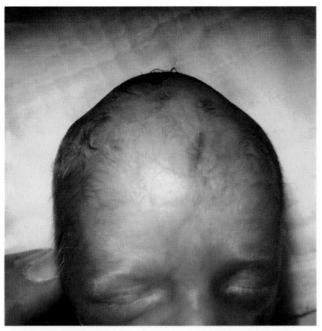

FIGURE 6–35. Intracranial hemorrhage—bulging fontanelle

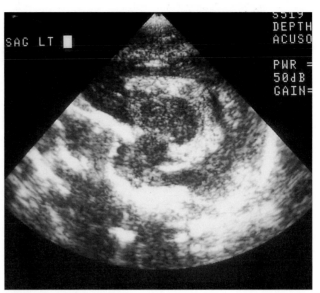

Intracranial Hemorrhage

FIGURE 6–37. Ultrasound: Grade III intraventricular hemorrhage, ventricular enlargement with blood

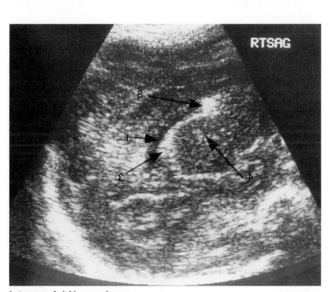

Intracranial Hemorrhage

FIGURE 6–36. Ultrasound: Grade I intraventricular subependymal hemorrhage

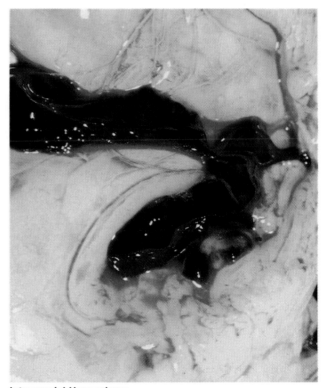

Intracranial Hemorrhage

FIGURE 6–38. Blood in lateral ventricle

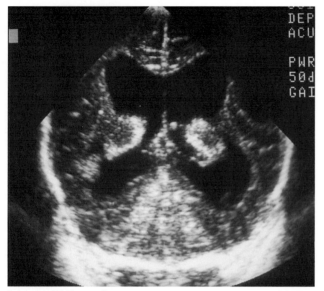

Intracranial Hemorrhage

FIGURE 6–39. Ultrasound: Grade IV intraventricular hemorrhage with parenchymal involvement

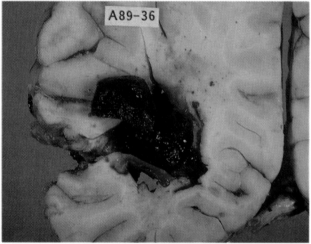

Intracranial Hemorrhage

FIGURE 6–40. Parenchymal hemorrhage

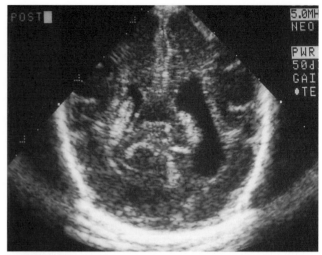

Intracranial Hemorrhage

FIGURE 6–41. Asymmetric ventricular enlargement

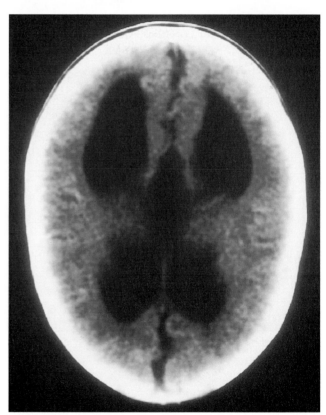

Intracranial Hemorrhage

FIGURE 6–42. Posthemorrhagic hydrocephalus

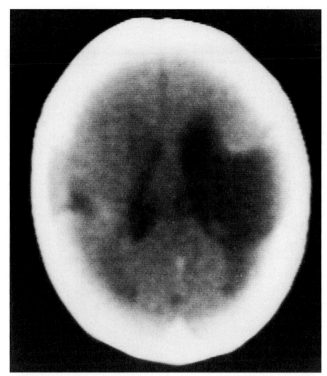

Intracranial Hemorrhage

FIGURE 6–43. Porencephalic cyst from parietal infarction

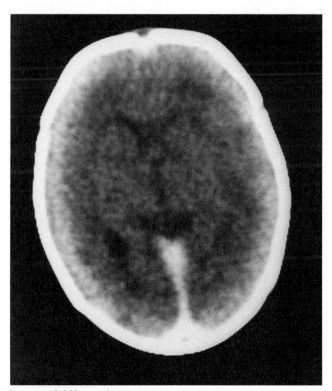

Intracranial Hemorrhage

FIGURE 6–44. Blood in the falx

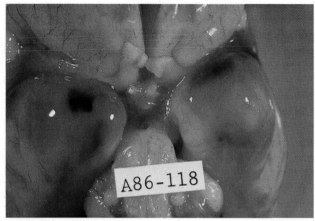

Intracranial Hemorrhage

FIGURE 6–45. Subarachnoid hemorrhage

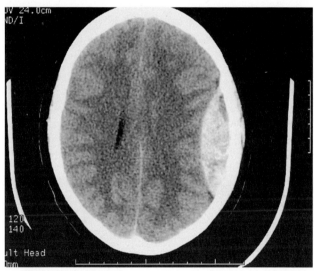

Intracranial Hemorrhage

FIGURE 6–46. Epidural hemorrhage, traumatic

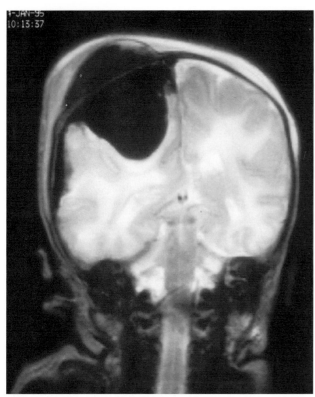

Intracranial Hemorrhage

FIGURE 6–47. MRI: subdural hemorrhage

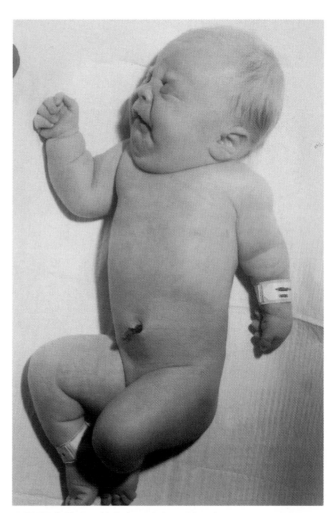

FIGURE 6–49. Brachial plexus injury, Erb palsy

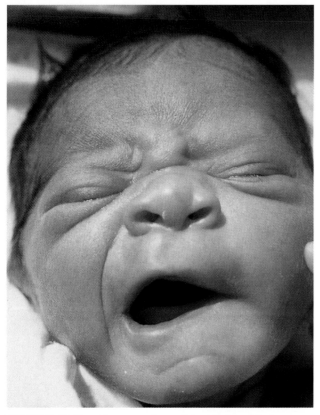

FIGURE 6–48. Seventh nerve palsy, unilateral facial paralysis

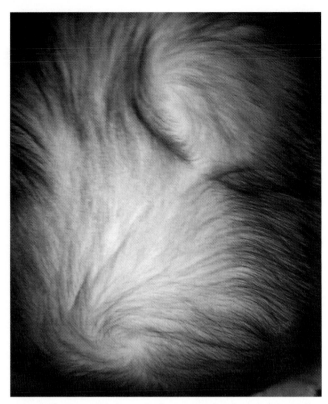

FIGURE 6–50. Double hair whorls associated with underlying malformed brain

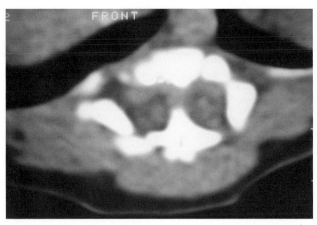

FIGURE 6–51. Diastematomyelia—the "double fried egg" appearance of a bisected spinal cord

SELECTED REFERENCES

Jones KL. (1997) Smith's Recognizable Patterns of Human Malformation. Philadelphia, WB Saunders.

Polin RA and Fox WW. (1998) Fetal and Neonatal Physiology. Philadelphia, WB Saunders, Chapters 78-94.

Taeusch HW and Ballard R. (1998) Avery's Diseases of the Newborn, 7th ed. Philadelphia, WB Saunders, Chapters 66-69.

Volpe J. (1995) Neurology of the Newborn, 3rd ed. Philadelphia, WB Saunders.

7 Otorhinolaryngology

Anomalies of the ear, nose, and palate are relatively common. They may be related to specific syndromes, especially major chromosomal abnormalities. However, any abnormality of the external ear increases the likelihood that the child will be hearing impaired. Approximately 25% of hearing loss are due to a genetic etiology. A significant portion is thought to be due to transplacental viral infection, especially unrecognized in utero cytomegalovirus infection. The five factors that are identified with a high potential for hearing impairment include a family history of childhood deafness, maternal viral infection, maxillofacial anomalies, hyperbilirubinemia, and a low birth weight, especially in those infants requiring intensive medical intervention.

Many of the oral findings are minor. However, cleft lip and cleft palate present significant problems with respect to feeding, respiratory and middle ear infections, and maternal attachment. Isolated cleft lip is distinct from isolated cleft palate. The fusion of the three mesodermal components to form the lip should occur by 5 weeks of gestation. In contrast, the fusion of the palate should be complete by 9 weeks' gestation. Approximately 50% of midfacial anomalies include both cleft lip and cleft palate. Twenty-five percent involve the palate only, and the remaining 25% involve the lip only. Cleft lip is bilateral in 20% of the cases, and there is a higher association of cleft palate in this subset. Many syndromes with multiple malformations have associated cleft lip and cleft palate. As many as 50% of children with both cleft lip and cleft palate have sufficient identifying features to describe a specific syndrome. Therefore, any newborn infant with major oral-facial anomalies requires a thorough evaluation for other associated congenital defects. Table 7-1 lists the developmental aspects of the nasopharynx and ear.

TABLE 7-1

DEVELOPMENT OF THE NASOPHARYNX AND EAR	
24 days	Otic placode
	Mandible
30 days	Otic invagination
34 days	Otic vesicle
	Olfactory placodes
38 days	Endolymph sac
	External auditory meatus
	Nasal swellings
44 days	Choana
52 days	Cochlea
8 wks	Ear canals
	Sublingual gland
10 wks	Lips
	Nasal cartilage
12 wks	Tonsillar crypts
16 wks	Cochlea differentiating
	Palate complete
	Teeth—enamel and dentine
20 wks	Inner ear ossified
	Ossification of nose
24 wks	Nares open
	Tooth primordia calcify
32 wks	Auricular cartilage
	Taste sense
1-2 mos	Salivary gland ducts canalize

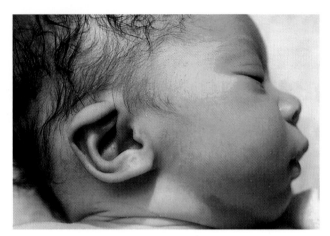

FIGURE 7–1. Low-set, posteriorly rotated auricle

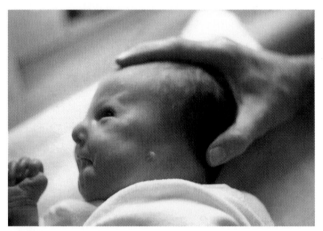

FIGURE 7–2. Microtia

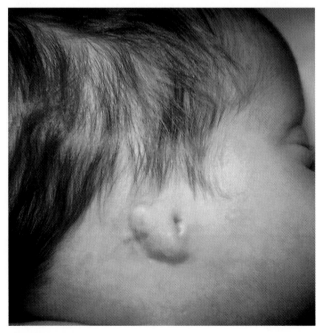

FIGURE 7–3. Hypoplastic auricle

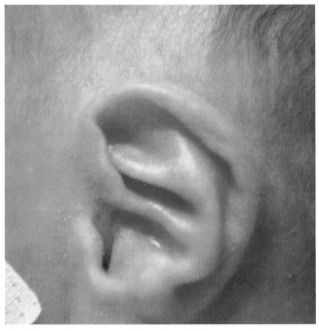

FIGURE 7–4. Redundant folding of cartilage

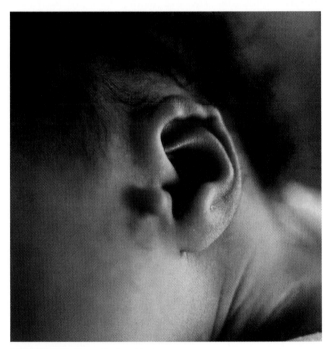

FIGURE 7–5. Preauricular skin tag

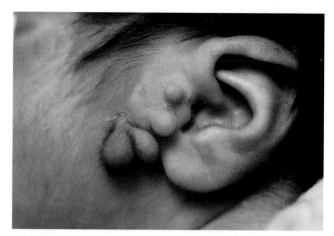

FIGURE 7–6. Multiple preauricular skin tags (Goldenhar syndrome)

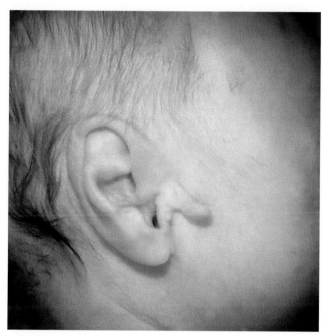

FIGURE 7–7. Preauricular cartilage horn

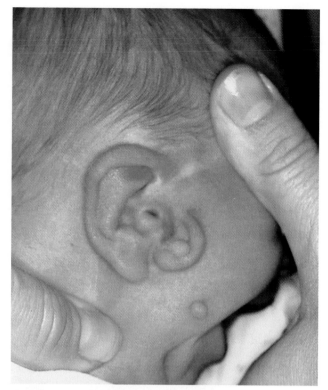

FIGURE 7–8. Duplication of cartilage

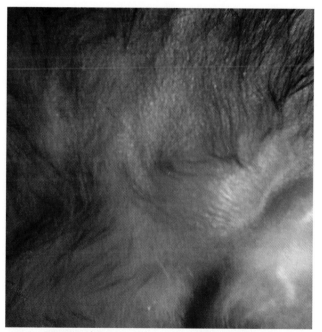

FIGURE 7–9. Postauricular cyst

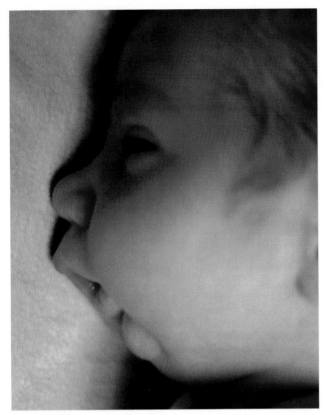

Micrognathia

FIGURE 7–10. Pierre Robin syndrome

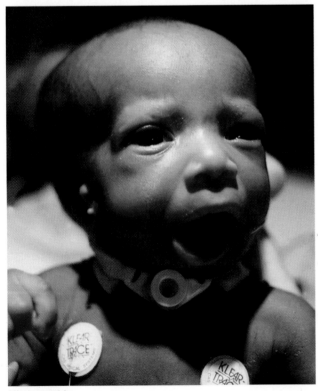

Micrognathia

FIGURE 7–11. Tracheostomy

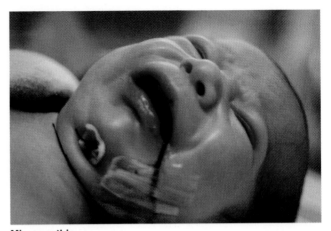

Micrognathia

FIGURE 7–12. Tongue button

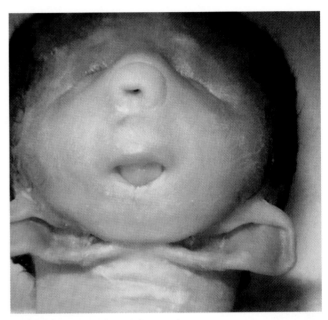

FIGURE 7–13. Branchial cleft anomaly

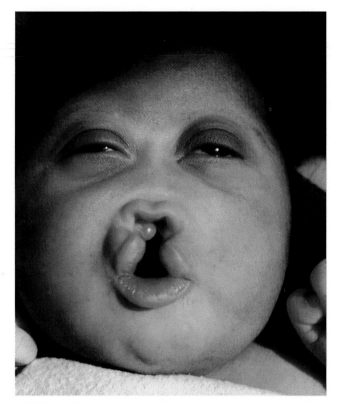

FIGURE 7–14. Holoprosencephaly

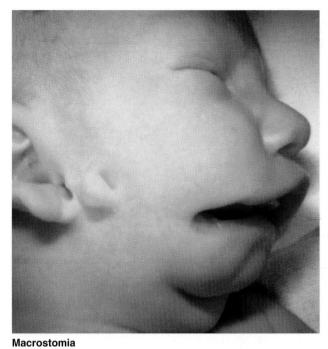

Macrostomia

FIGURE 7–16. Profile

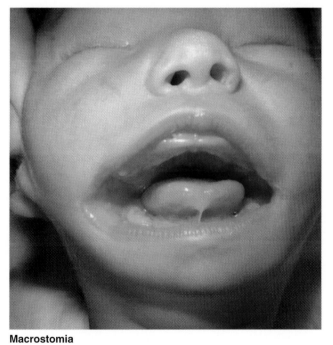

Macrostomia

FIGURE 7–15. En face

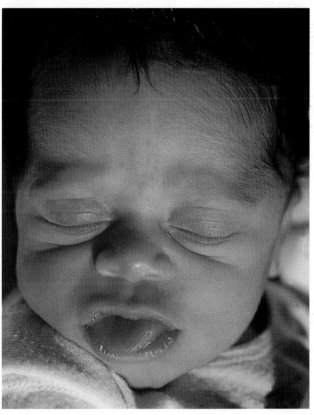

FIGURE 7–17. Macroglossia

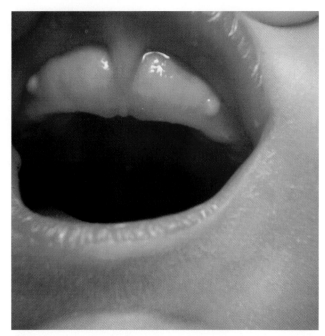

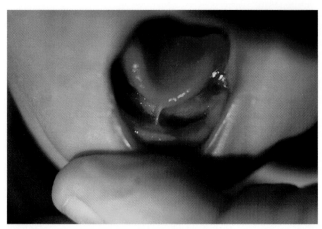

FIGURE 7–20. Ankyloglossia inferior (tongue-tie)

FIGURE 7–18. Bohn nodules

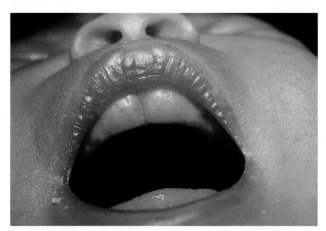

FIGURE 7–19. Gingival hyperplasia due to chronic maternal hydantoin therapy

NEONATAL TEETH

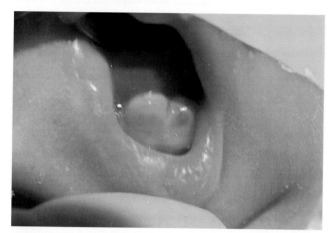

FIGURE 7–21. Tooth eruption cyst

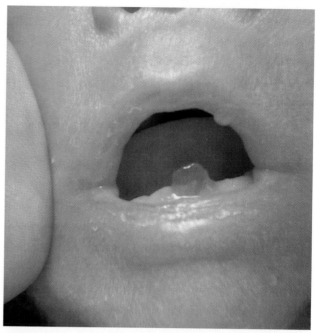

FIGURE 7–23. False tooth cap removed, leaving residual tissue

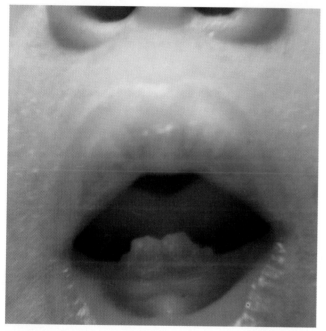

FIGURE 7–22. True teeth with roots

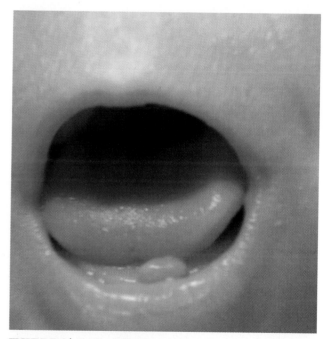

FIGURE 7–24. Epulis of gingiva

NOSE

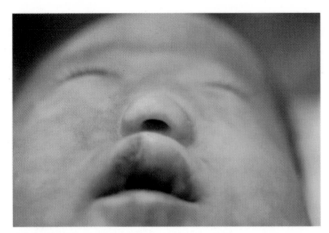

FIGURE 7–25. Single nostril—holoprosencephaly

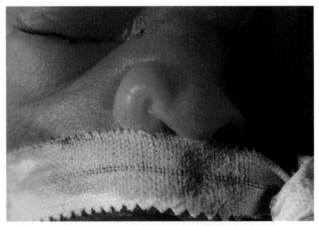

FIGURE 7–26. Duplicated nostril

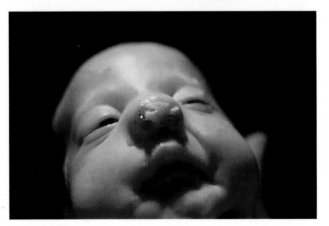

FIGURE 7–27. Defective cartilage of the tip of the nose

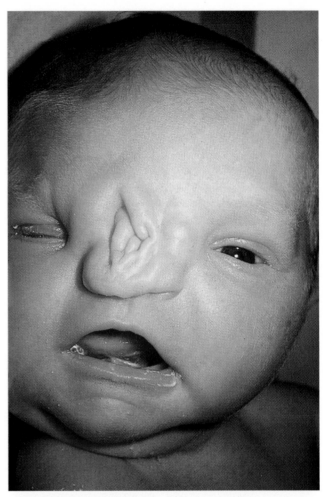

FIGURE 7–28. Frontonasal dysplasia

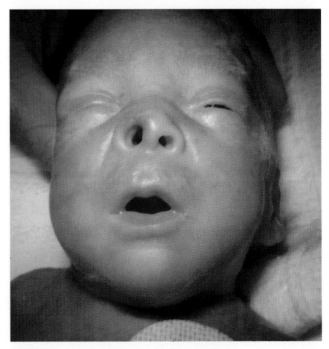

FIGURE 7–29. Enlarged nostril from intubation

CHOANAL ATRESIA

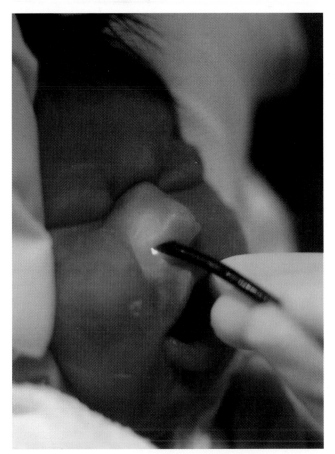

FIGURE 7–30. Fiberoptic scope examination of patency

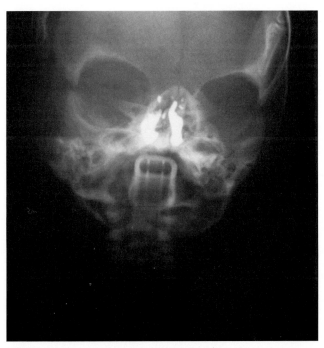

FIGURE 7–31. Anteroposterior radiograph with contrast material

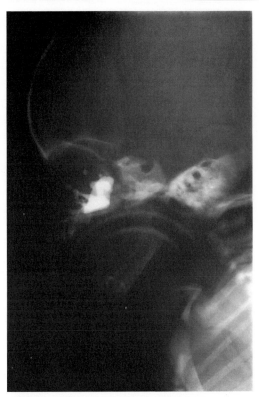

FIGURE 7–32. Lateral radiograph with contrast material

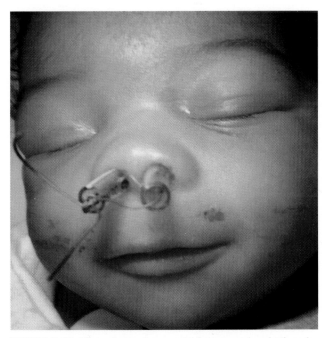

FIGURE 7–33. Bilateral nasopharyngeal tubes secured on both ends of the septum

POLYP

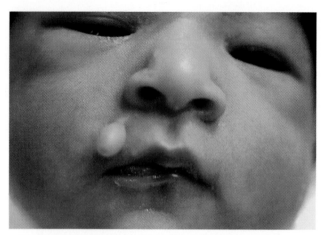

FIGURE 7–34. Paranasal polyp

LIP

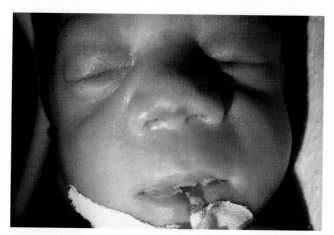

FIGURE 7–35. Long philtrum

CLEFT LIP

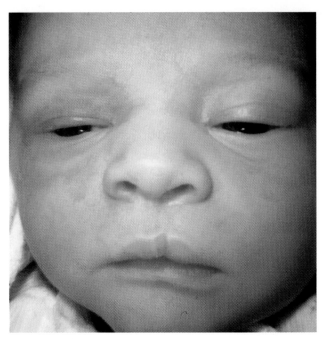

FIGURE 7–36. Aborted cleft lip

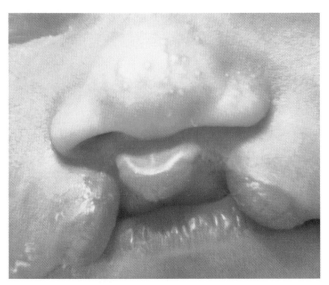

FIGURE 7–38. Bilateral cleft lip

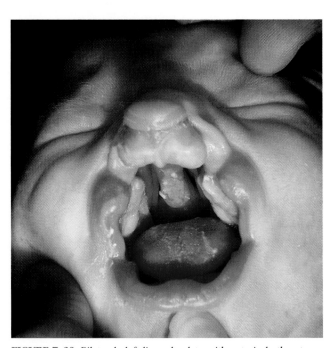

FIGURE 7–39. Bilateral cleft lip and palate with anteriorly thrust maxillary segment

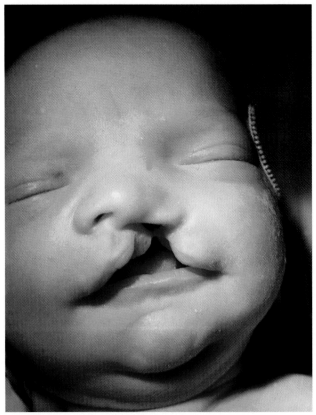

FIGURE 7–37. Unilateral cleft lip

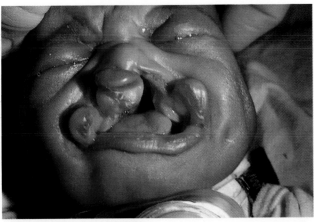

Massive Cleft Lip and Palate

FIGURE 7–40. At birth

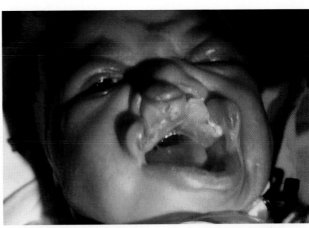

Massive Cleft Lip and Palate

FIGURE 7–42. Prosthesis in place, creating an artificial palate

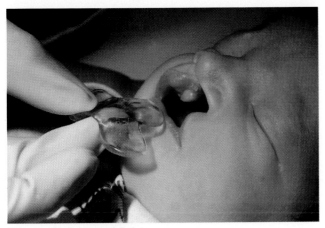

Massive Cleft Lip and Palate

FIGURE 7–41. Prosthesis insertion

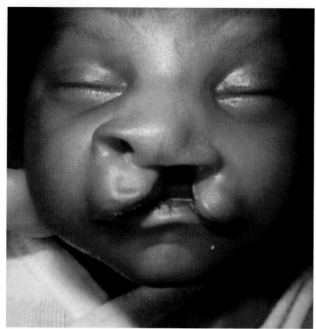

Cleft Lip with Nasal Deformity

FIGURE 7–43. Preoperative

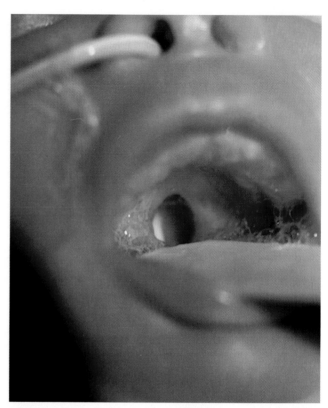

FIGURE 7–45. Isolated cleft of soft palate

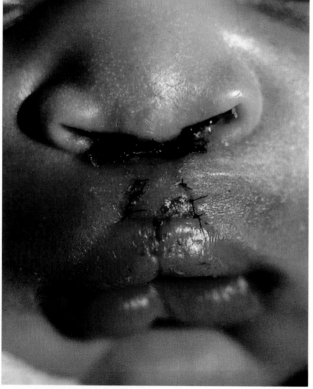

Cleft Lip with Nasal Deformity

FIGURE 7–44. Postoperative, with alignment of vermilion border

ECTOPIA

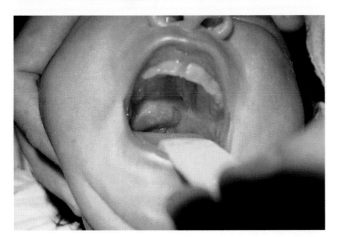

FIGURE 7–46. Ectopic brain on palate

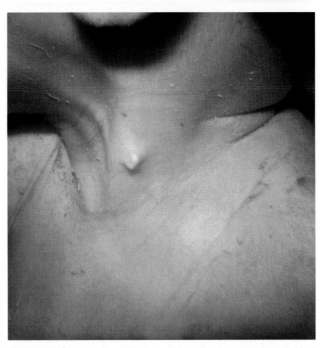

FIGURE 7–47. Ectopic cartilage overlying the sternocleidomastoid muscle

DUCT

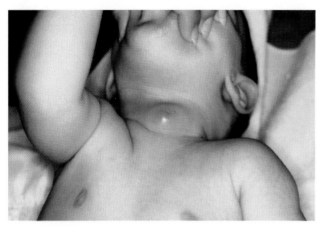

FIGURE 7–48. Infected thyroglossal duct cyst

LARYNX AND TRACHEA

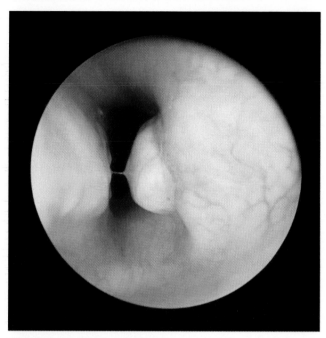

FIGURE 7–49. Vocal cord granuloma

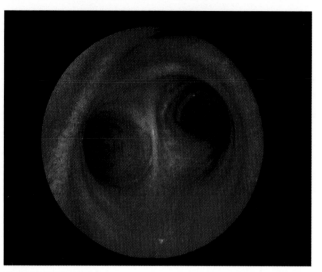

FIGURE 7–51. Carina

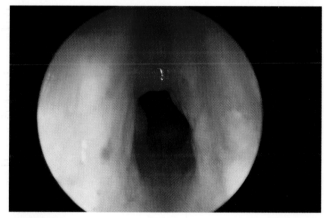

FIGURE 7–50. Subglottic stenosis

SELECTED REFERENCES

Jones KL. (1997) Smith's Recognizable Patterns of Human Malformation, 5th ed. Philadelphia, WB Saunders.

Kenner C, Brueggemeyer A, and Gunderson LP, Eds. (1993) Comprehensive Neonatal Nursing. Philadelphia, WB Saunders, Chapters 17 and 18.

Moore KL and Persaud TVN. (1993) The Developing Human, 5th ed. Philadelphia, WB Saunders.

Polin RA and Fox WW. (1998) Fetal and Neonatal Physiology, 2nd ed. Philadelphia, WB Saunders, Chapter 201.

Taeusch HW and Ballard RA. (1998) Avery's Diseases of the Newborn, 7th ed. Philadelphia, WB Saunders, Chapters 20, 71.

8 Gastrointestinal

The primary function of the intestinal tract is to provide a large surface area sufficient for digestion, absorption, and excretion. In addition, the intestinal mucosa provides a barrier containing the noxious substances within the lumen. The increase in the surface area of the intestine to allow efficient absorption results from formation of villi from the stratified epithelium and subsequently dense microvilli. Table 8–1 outlines some of the important developmental aspects of the maturation of the intestinal tract.

Intestinal crypts and villi are found in the human fetal intestine by 10 to 12 weeks of gestation, with a progressive development from proximal to distal intestine. The morphologic development of the intestine is nearly complete by 22 weeks' gestation. The microvillous membrane of the columnar epithelial cells becomes the primary location of digestion and absorption, with progressive maturation of intestinal enzymes from the second trimester of fetal development through postnatal life.

Most of the peptidases are present by 22 weeks' gestation. These allow relatively efficient digestion of the whey-like proteins swallowed from amniotic fluid. Amino acid transport has been demonstrated in the fetal intestine within the second trimester. The digestion of lipid is inefficient in neonates because of low bile salt pools and poor reabsorption of bile salts in the distal ileum. In addition, there are low levels of intestinal and pancreatic lipases in the preterm newborn infant. Active transport of glucose occurs as early as 11 weeks' gestation and will reach two thirds of the adult value by 21 weeks' gestation.

The enteric nervous system is complex and matures paralleling the development of the central nervous system. The coordination of a mature sucking reflex to swallow occurs at approximately 34 weeks' gestation. The majority of preterm infants have poor intestinal motility along with mixed nutrient malabsorption, two conditions which predispose them to necrotizing enterocolitis.

The following series of photographs include congenital defects that occur very early in gestation and some of the more common acquired conditions.

TABLE 8–1

DEVELOPMENT OF THE GASTROINTESTINAL SYSTEM

GESTATIONAL AGE (Wks)	CHARACTERISTICS
3.5	Separation of gut from yolk sac
5–6	Gallbladder forms Hepatic ducts appear Spleen
5–8	Circular muscle develops in small intestine
7.5	Fusion of pancreas
8	Gastric pits appear Intestinal villi Anal membrane ruptures
9–10	Colonic circular muscle
10	Longitudinal muscle forms in small intestine Intestine withdraws into the abdomen
12	Bile Primitive parietal cells Pancreatic islets Complete innervation of ganglion cells of the myenteric plexus
16	Meconium begins to fill the colon
22	Amylase detectable
22	Gastric glands mature
24–30	Rapid elongation and maturation
28	Single sucks
31	Sucking bursts
34	Mature sucks, coordination with swallowing

TRACHEOESOPHAGEAL (TE) FISTULA

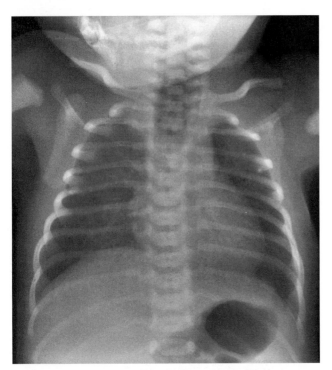

FIGURE 8–1. TE fistula, esophageal pouch

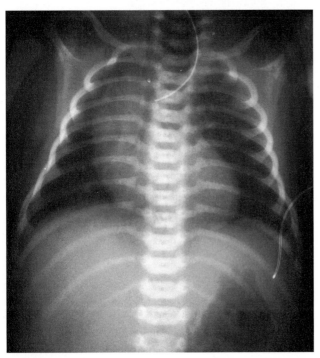

FIGURE 8–2. TE fistula, nasogastric tube in pouch

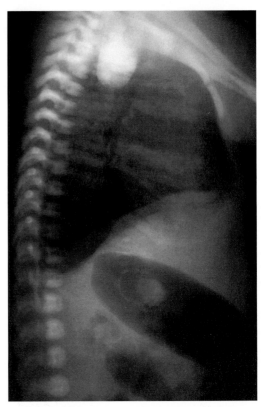

FIGURE 8–3. Lateral view contrast in pouch

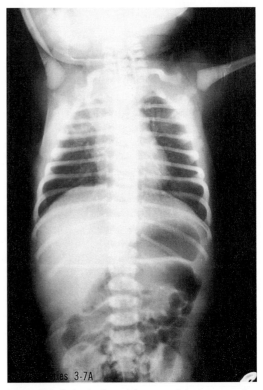

FIGURE 8–4. Aspiration, right upper lobe pneumonia

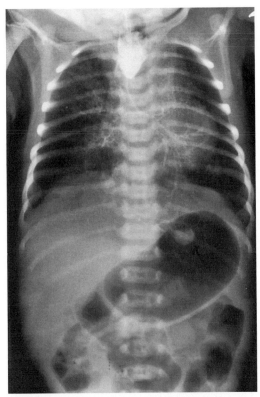

FIGURE 8–5. Bronchogram from aspiration of contrast material unnecessarily instilled into the esophageal pouch

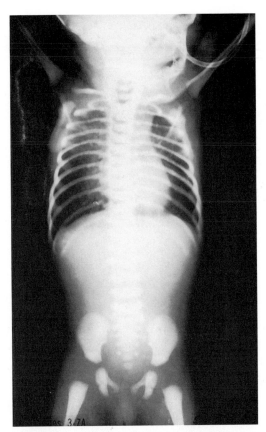

FIGURE 8–7. Proximal TE fistula—no distal fistula with airless abdomen

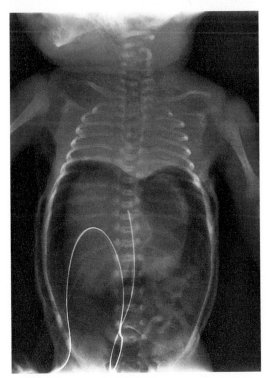

FIGURE 8–6. Pneumoperitoneum from ruptured TE fistula and paraesophageal dissection

ESOPHAGEAL ATRESIA WITHOUT TE FISTULA

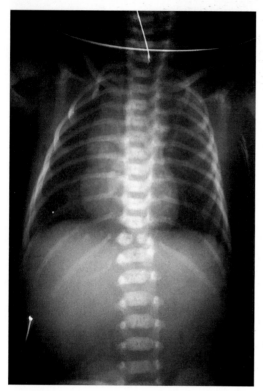

FIGURE 8–8. Anteroposterior view

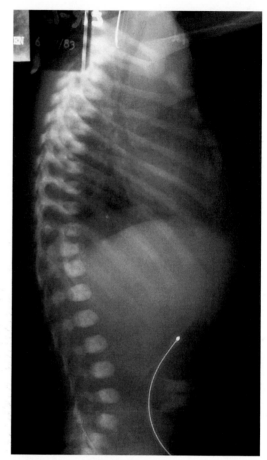

FIGURE 8–9. Lateral view

ESOPHAGUS

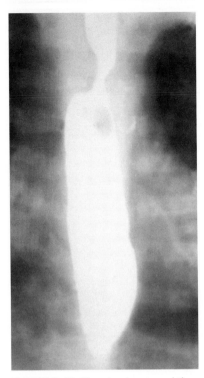

FIGURE 8–10. Vascular ring around the esophagus

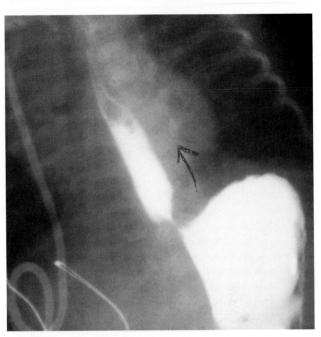

FIGURE 8–11. Gastroesophageal reflux *(arrow)*

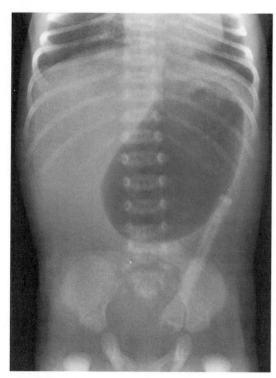

FIGURE 8–12. Pyloric atresia—single bubble

PYLORIC STENOSIS

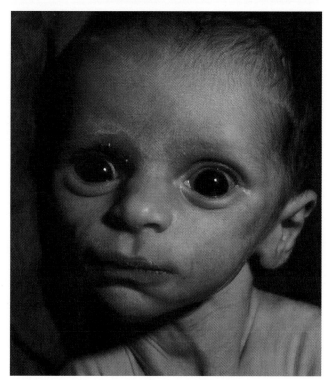

FIGURE 8–13. Two week old infant: dehydration from recurrent vomiting

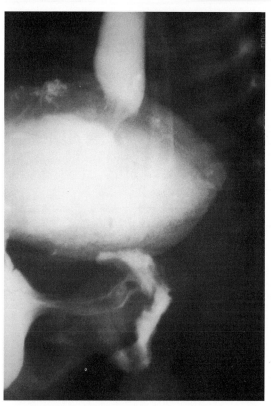

FIGURE 8–14. Radiographic string sign of contrast material in severely narrowed segment

DUODENAL ATRESIA

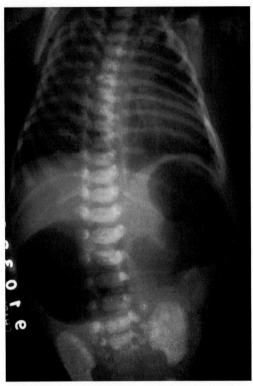

FIGURE 8–15. Double bubble

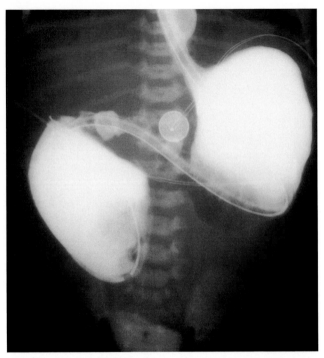

FIGURE 8–16. Double bubble with contrast

ANNULAR PANCREAS

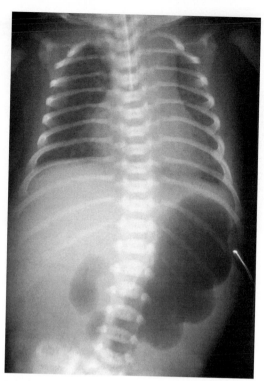

FIGURE 8–17. Radiograph: intestinal obstruction

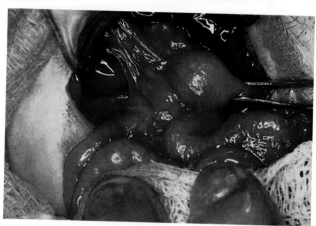

FIGURE 8–18. Intraoperative view

JEJUNAL ATRESIA

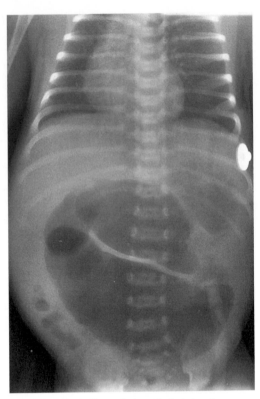

FIGURE 8–19. Radiograph: intestinal obstruction

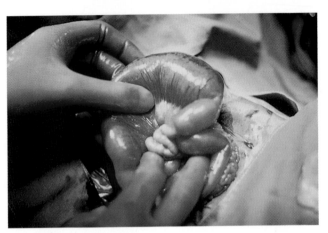

FIGURE 8–20. Intraoperative view

ILEAL ATRESIA

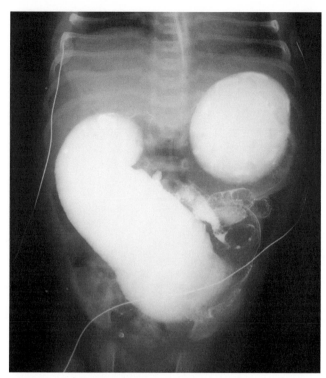

FIGURE 8–21. Radiograph: distal obstruction

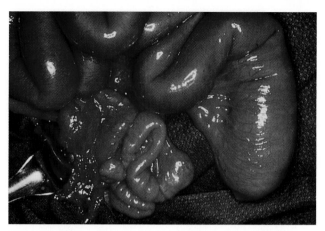

FIGURE 8–23. Proximal intestinal dilation with distal small caliber

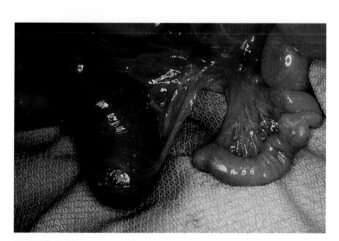

FIGURE 8–22. Intraoperative view

COLON

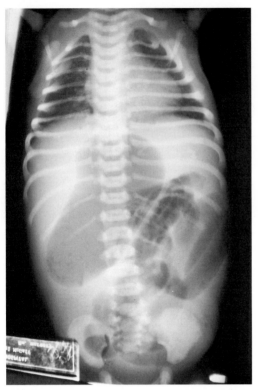

FIGURE 8–24. Colonic atresia

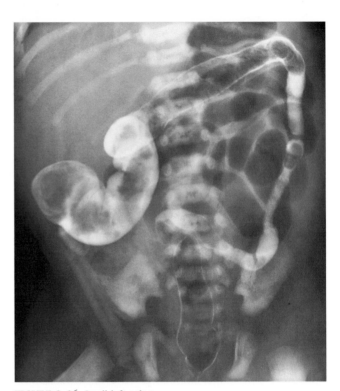

FIGURE 8–26. Small left colon

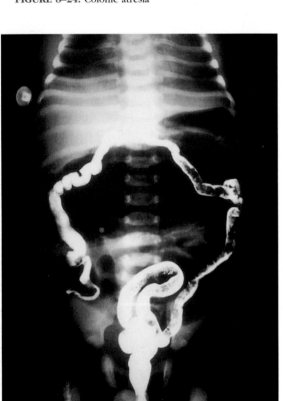

FIGURE 8–25. Microcolon

VOLVULUS

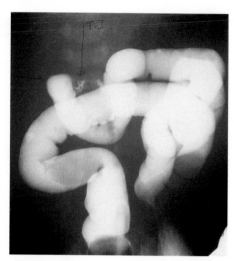

FIGURE 8–27. Barium enema: colon malpositioned

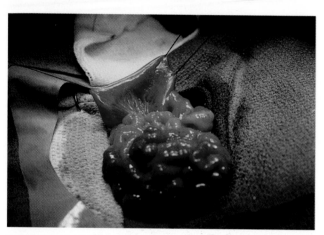

FIGURE 8–29. Viable bowel at surgery

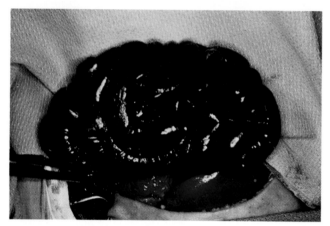

FIGURE 8–28. Necrotic bowel in surgery

INTUSSUSCEPTION

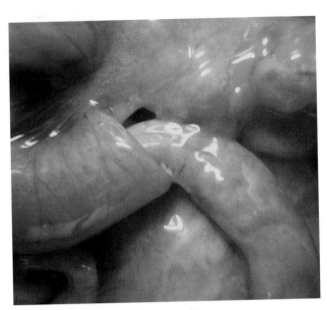

FIGURE 8–30. Small bowel, intraoperative

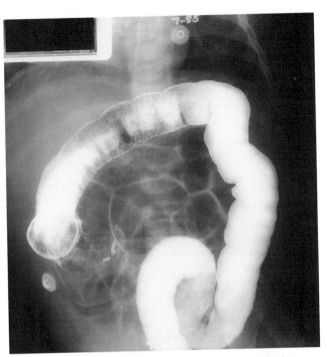

FIGURE 8–32. Radiograph: barium enema to reduce a colonic intussusception

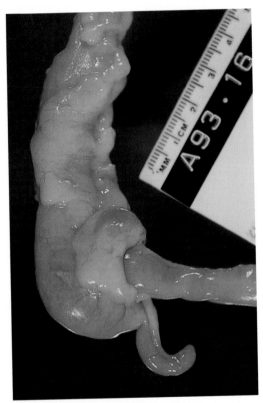

FIGURE 8–31. Ileocolonic, postmortem

IMPERFORATE ANUS

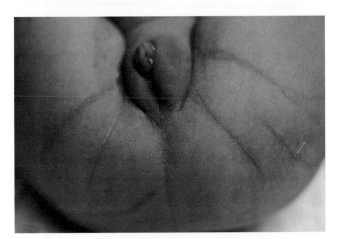

FIGURE 8–33. Anal sphincter absent

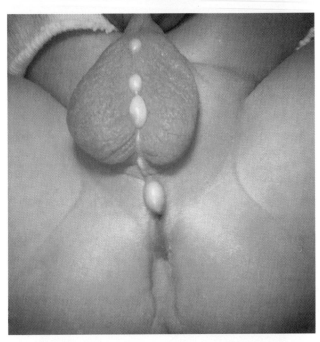

FIGURE 8–35. Perineal fistula with segmentation of leading mucous plug

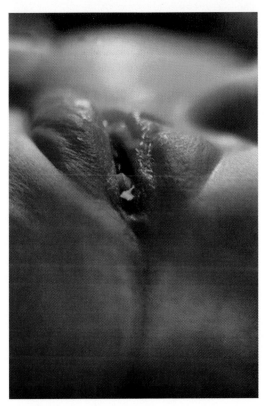

FIGURE 8–34. Anal sphincter tone present

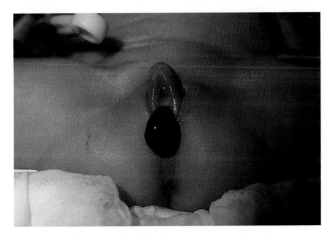

FIGURE 8–36. Rectovaginal fistula

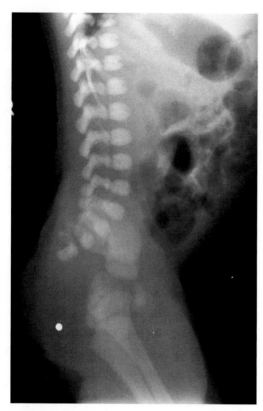

FIGURE 8–37. Lateral radiograph with metal dot on skin over imperforation

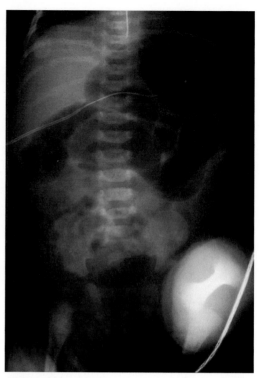

FIGURE 8–38. Radiograph: multiple distended loops of large and small bowel

MECONIUM

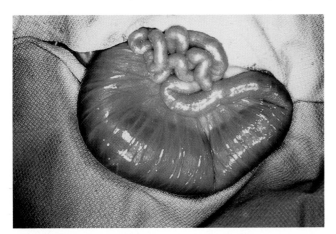

FIGURE 8–39. Meconium ileus

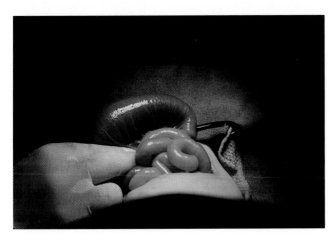

FIGURE 8–40. Meconium plug, cystic fibrosis, intraoperative view

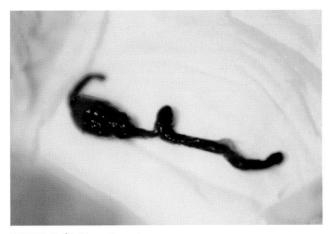

FIGURE 8–41. Meconium plug

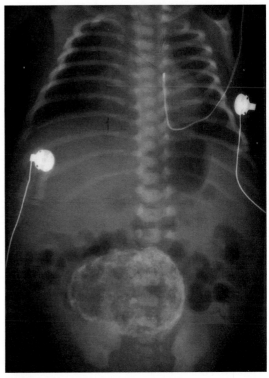

FIGURE 8–42. Anteroposterior radiograph—calcified meconium cyst

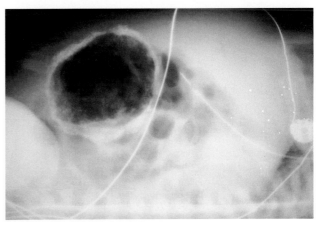

FIGURE 8–43. Lateral radiograph—calcified meconium cyst

DIVERTICULUM

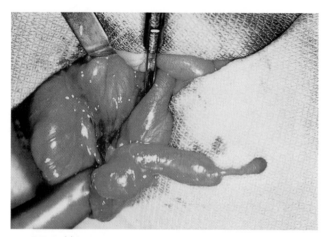

FIGURE 8–44. Meckel's diverticulum

HERNIATION

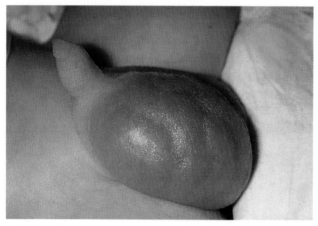

FIGURE 8–45. Inguinal hernia with bowel in the scrotum

RECTAL PROLAPSE

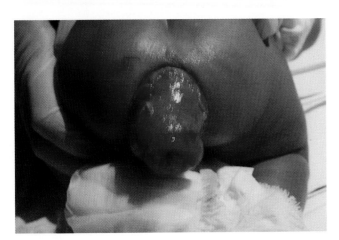

FIGURE 8–46. Cystic fibrosis

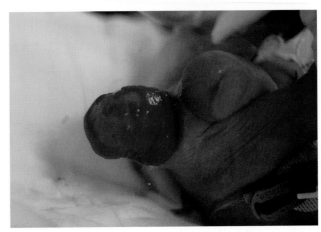

FIGURE 8–47. Preterm baby—chronic lung disease and increased intra-abdominal pressure

LACTOBEZOAR

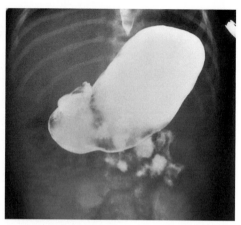

FIGURE 8–48. Radiolucent stomach mass surrounded by contrast material. The preterm baby was unable to digest the casein-based formula.

POLYSPLENIA

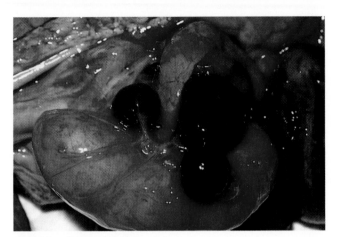

FIGURE 8–49. Polysplenia

ASCITES

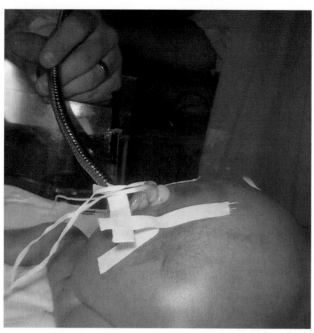

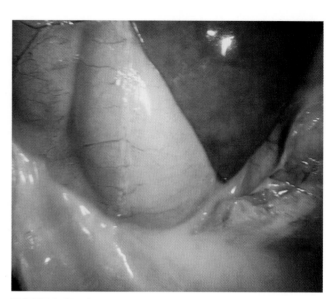

FIGURE 8–52. Chylous ascites

FIGURE 8–50. Gross abdominal distention with congenital ascites

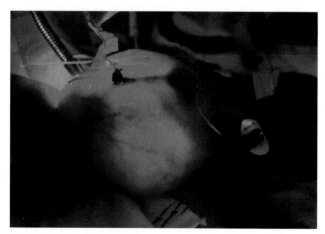

FIGURE 8–51. Transillumination

STOOL

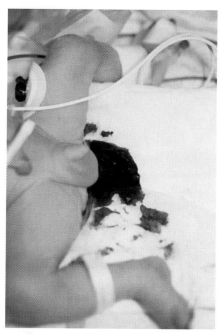

FIGURE 8–53. Bloody stool: swallowed maternal blood

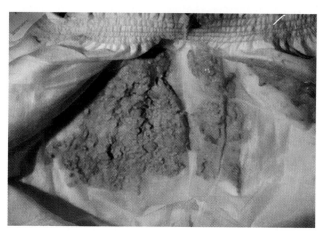

FIGURE 8–55. Pale stool: congenital hepatitis

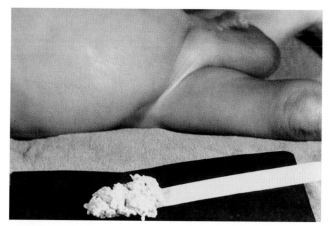

FIGURE 8–54. Pale stool: biliary atresia with associated jaundice

PORTAL HYPERTENSION

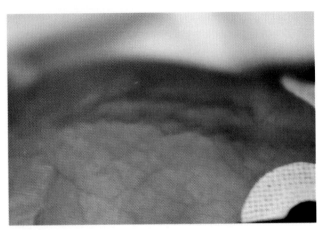

FIGURE 8–56. Cutaneous vascular shunt

HIRSCHSPRUNG DISEASE

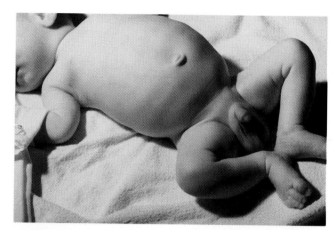

FIGURE 8–57. Abdominal distention with visible bowel loops

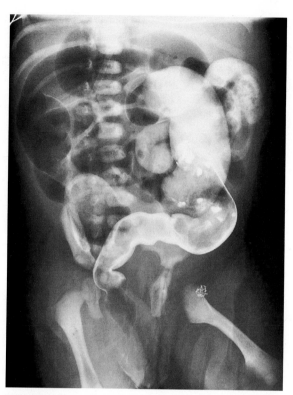

FIGURE 8–59. Radiograph: barium enema demonstrating a narrowed rectal segment

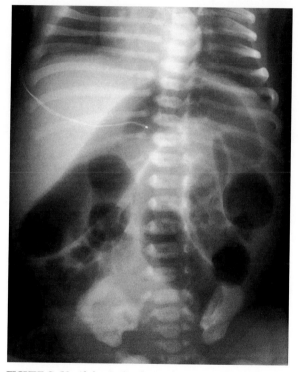

FIGURE 8–58. Abdominal radiograph: gaseous distention of bowel loops indicating obstruction

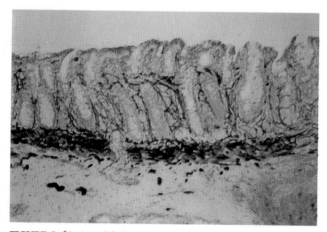

FIGURE 8–60. Acetylcholinesterase stain consistent with an absence of ganglion cells

NECROTIZING ENTEROCOLITIS

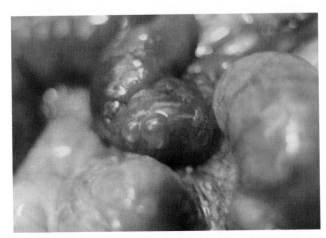

FIGURE 8–61. Pneumatosis intestinalis

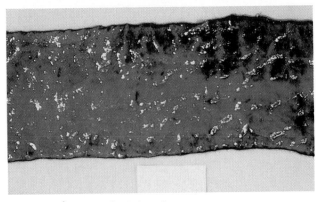

FIGURE 8–62. Hemorrhagic intestine

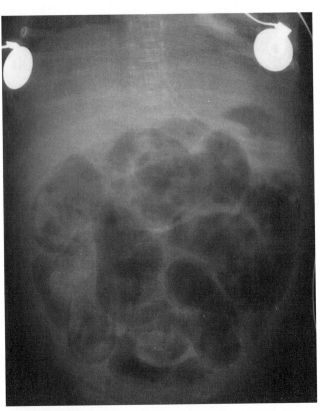

FIGURE 8–63. Right lower quadrant pneumatosis

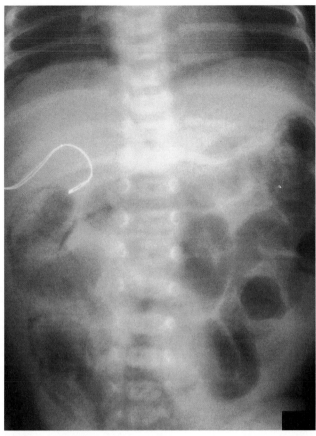

FIGURE 8–64. Diffuse pneumatosis

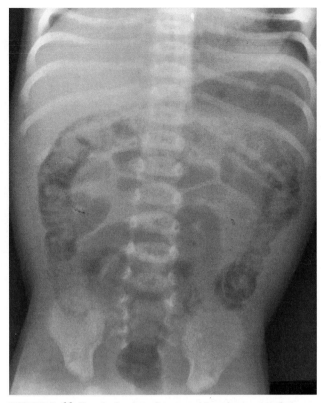

FIGURE 8–66. Sloughed colon after a partial exchange transfusion for polycythemia

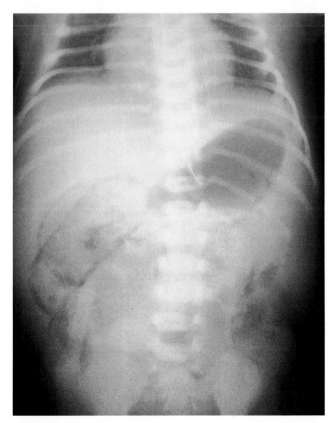

FIGURE 8–65. Colonic pneumatosis

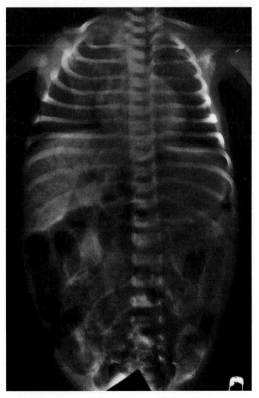

FIGURE 8–67. Pneumatosis and diffuse portal air

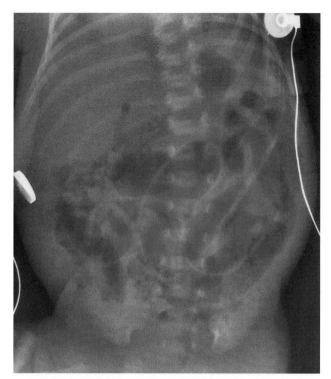

FIGURE 8–68. Distended bowel loops and portal air

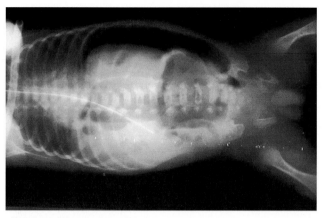

FIGURE 8–70. Decubitus—free abdominal air

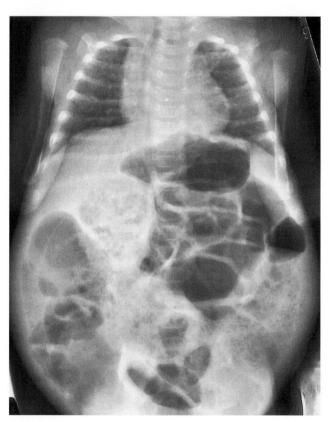

FIGURE 8–71. Intestinal obstruction due to multiple strictures and adhesions

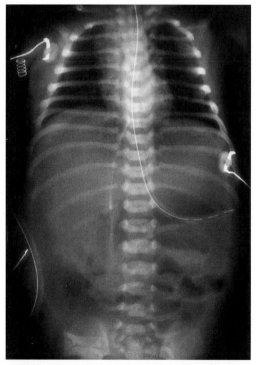

FIGURE 8–69. Pneumoperitoneum—falciform ligament evident

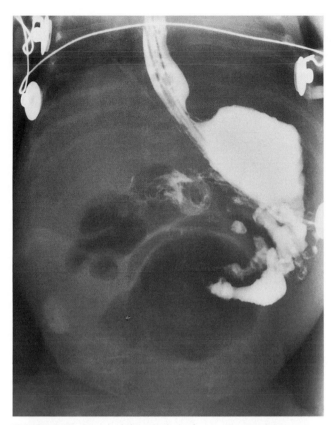

FIGURE 8–72. Intestinal diverticulum after acute necrotizing enterocolitis

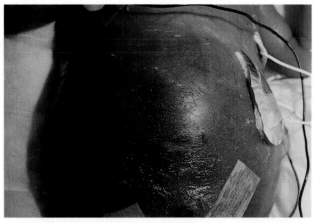

FIGURE 8–73. Peritonitis—discolored abdomen

ABDOMINAL WALL DEFECTS

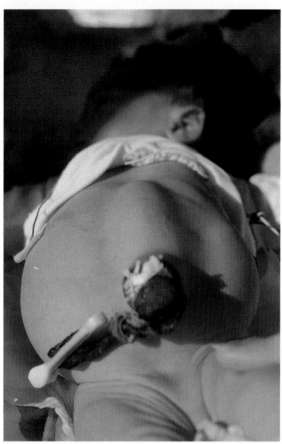

FIGURE 8–74. Diastasis recti abdominis

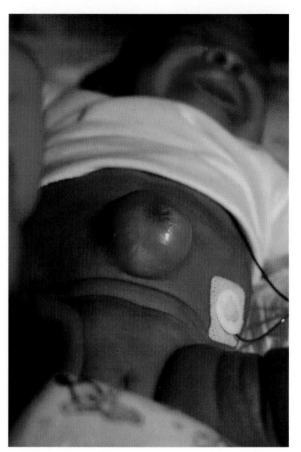

FIGURE 8–75. Umbilical hernia

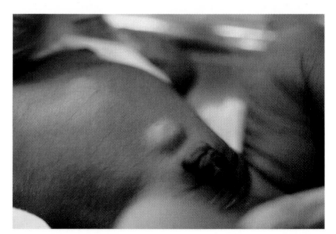

FIGURE 8–76. Richter hernia

PRUNE-BELLY SYNDROME (TRIAD SYNDROME)

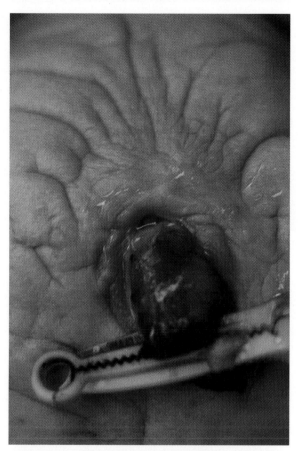

FIGURE 8–77. Minimal abdominal musculature with redundant lax skin

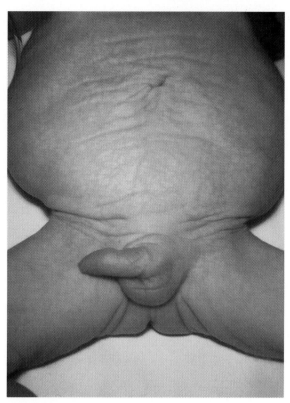

FIGURE 8–78. Undescended testes

OMPHALOCELE

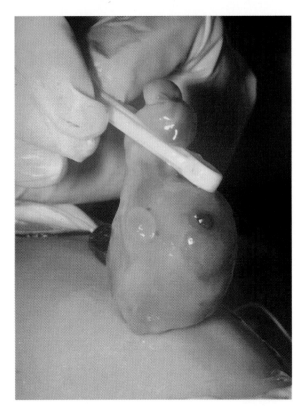

FIGURE 8–79. Small, intact sac at the base of the umbilical cord

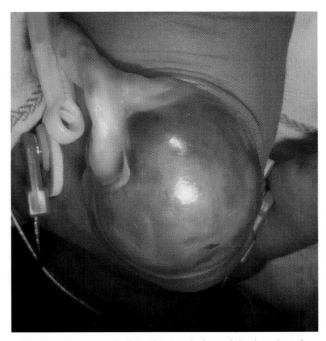

FIGURE 8–80. Intact, thickened sac with the umbilical cord on the surface

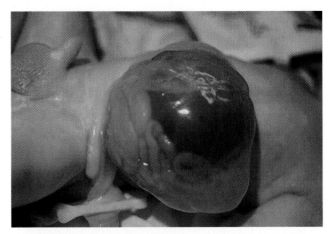

FIGURE 8–81. Intact sac with healthy organs visible

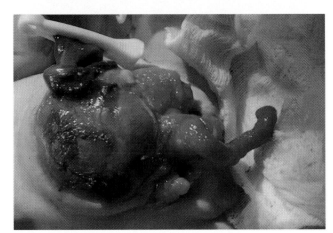

FIGURE 8–82. Intrauterine rupture of the sac with bowel necrosis

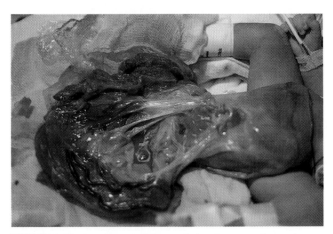

FIGURE 8–83. Attachment of the omphalocele sac to placental membranes

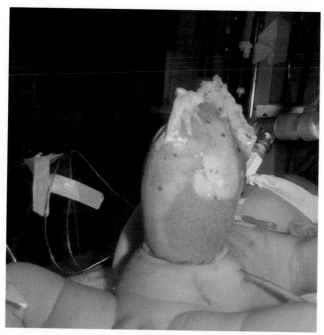

FIGURE 8–84. Chimney closure of an omphalocele

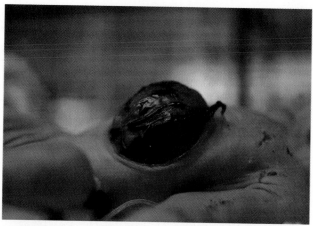

FIGURE 8–85. Granulation of the omphalocele sac in a baby with inoperable congenital heart disease

GASTROSCHISIS

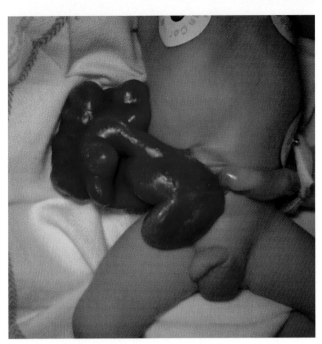

FIGURE 8–86. Thickened, matted bowel loops

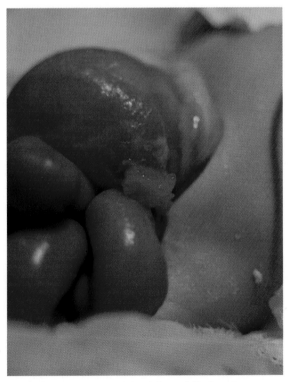

FIGURE 8–87. Distinct origin of the umbilical cord

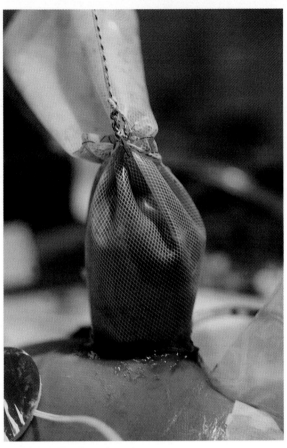

FIGURE 8–88. Silastic bag closure

SELECTED REFERENCES

Gryboski J. (1975) Gastrointestinal Problems in the Infant. Philadelphia, WB Saunders.

Jones KL. (1997) Smiths's Recognizable Patterns of Human Malformation. Philadelphia, WB Saunders.

McCullum LL and Thigpen JL. Assessment and management of gastrointestinal dysfunction. *In* Kenner C, Brueggemeyer A and Gunderson LP, Eds. (1993) Comprehensive Neonatal Nursing. Philadelphia, WB Saunders, pp 434–479.

Polin R and Fox WW. (1998) Fetal and Neonatal Physiology. Philadelphia, WB Saunders, Chapters 121–129.

Taeusch HW and Ballard RA. (1998) Avery's Diseases of the Newborn. Philadelphia, WB Saunders, Chapters 72–76.

9 Renal and Genitourinary

The genitourinary system can be divided into its two separate functional components: the urinary tract, which is excretory, and the genital tract, which is reproductive. Developmentally and anatomically, these systems are obviously very closely associated. Both the urinary tract and the gonads develop from intermediate mesoderm that extends along the dorsal aspect of the embryo. Table 9–1 summarizes the developmental progression of nephrogenesis.

Three sets of excretory organs develop in the human embryo: the pronephros, the mesonephros, and the

TABLE 9–1

DEVELOPMENT OF THE UROGENITAL TRACT

24 days	Mesonephric ridge
30 days	Mesonephric duct enters cloaca
34 days	Ureteral evagination
	Urorectal septation
38 days	Paramesonephric duct
7.5 wks	Renal vesicles
8 wks	Early glomeruli
	Fusion of müllerian ducts
10 wks	Renal excretion
	Bladder sac
	Urogenital sinus—müllerian tubes connect
12 wks	Regression of genital ducts
16 wks	Mesonephros involuting
	Uterus and vagina
	Kidney typical
40 wks +	Elongation of tubules
	Countercurrent concentrating gradient in loop of Henle

TABLE 9–2

INCIDENCE OF GENITOURINARY DEFECTS

Renal agenesis	
Unilateral	1/1000
Bilateral	3/1000
Ectopic kidney	1/700
Horseshoe kidney	1/500
Multicystic dysplasia	1/4300
Polycystic kidney disease (autosomal recessive)	1/10,000
Polycystic kidney disease (autosomal dominant)	1/3500

metanephros. The pronephros is not functional, whereas the mesonephros functions for a very short time during the early fetal period. The metanephros begins to produce urine by the end of the first trimester.

Approximately 10% of newborn infants have a congenital abnormality of the urinary tract. However, many of these are minor and do not interfere with function and therefore may not be discovered. A number of external characteristics have been associated with congenital renal anomalies: these include polydactyly and syndactyly, small mandibles, anorectal anomalies, and neural tube defects. Anomalies of the genitourinary systems are particularly common in gross chromosomal malformations. The incidence of some of the more common forms of renal disease is presented in Table 9–2.

The remainder of the photographs in this section primarily show mild developmental abnormalities that are not life-threatening and are easily corrected.

RENAL AGENESIS—OLIGOHYDRAMNIOS

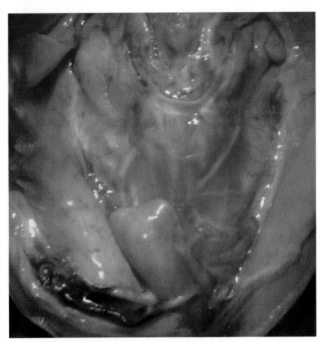

FIGURE 9–1. Abdomen: absent kidneys

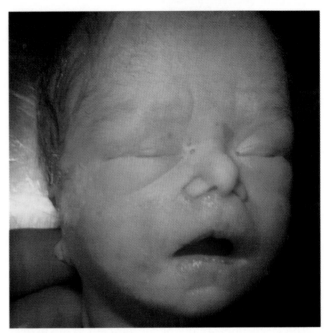

FIGURE 9–3. Facial flattening

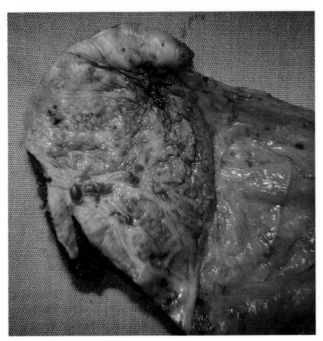

FIGURE 9–2. Placenta: amnion nodosum

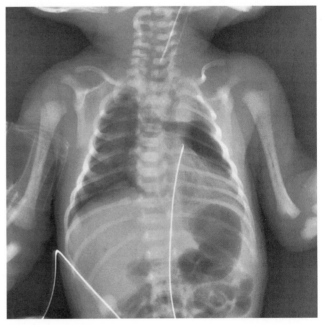

FIGURE 9–4. Pulmonary hypoplasia

POLYCYSTIC KIDNEYS—OLIGOHYDRAMNIOS SEQUENCE

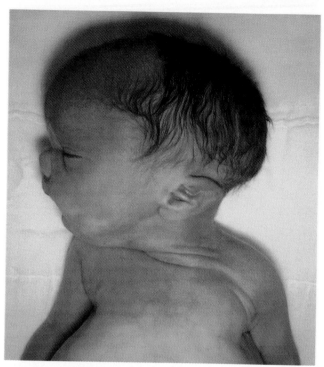

FIGURE 9–5. Facial compression

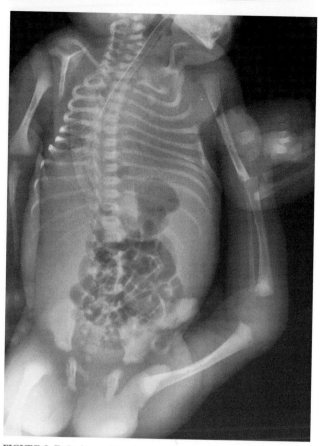

FIGURE 9–7. Radiograph: pulmonary hypoplasia and large abdominal masses pushing the gas-filled intestine centrally

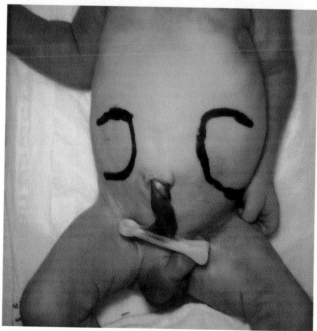

FIGURE 9–6. Bilateral flank masses

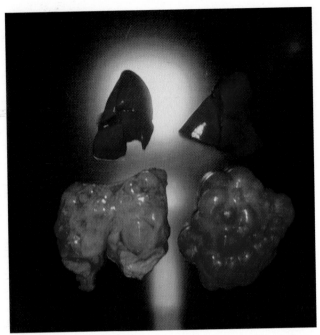

FIGURE 9–8. Gross pathology: small lungs with cystic kidneys

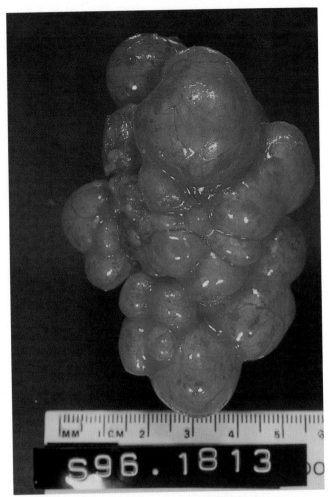

FIGURE 9–9. Polycystic kidney (autosomal dominant)

MULTICYSTIC DYSPLASTIC KIDNEY

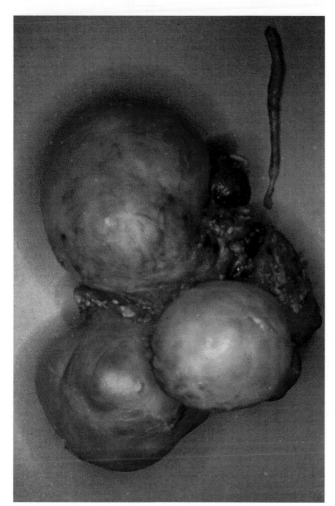

FIGURE 9–10. Gross specimen

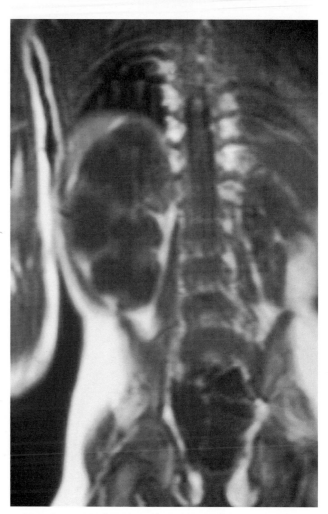

FIGURE 9–11. MRI demonstrating multiple renal cysts

POTTER CLASSIFICATION OF RENAL CYSTIC DISEASE

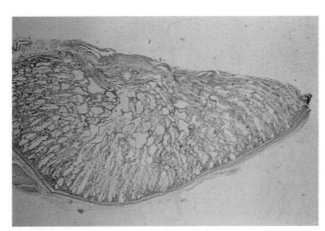

Type I Autosomal Recessive Polycystic Kidney

FIGURE 9–12. Scanning view, diffuse small cysts

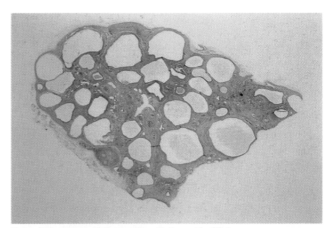

Type II Autosomal Recessive Polycystic Kidney

FIGURE 9–14. Scanning view, peripheral large cysts

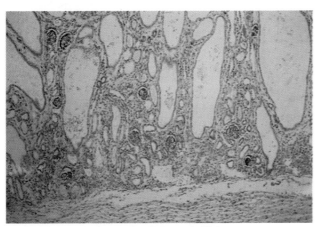

Type I Autosomal Recessive Polycystic Kidney

FIGURE 9–13. Detailed view

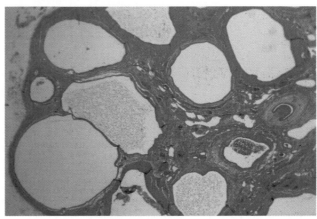

Type II Autosomal Recessive Polycystic Kidney

FIGURE 9–15. Detailed view

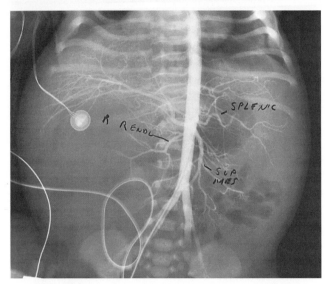

FIGURE 9–16. Large right renal cyst demonstrated as a filling defect by an arteriogram

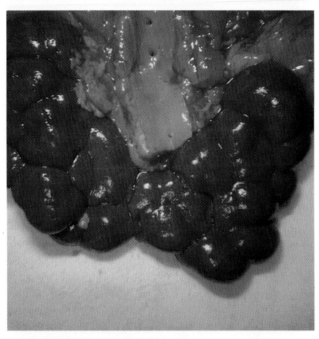

FIGURE 9–18. Horseshoe kidney

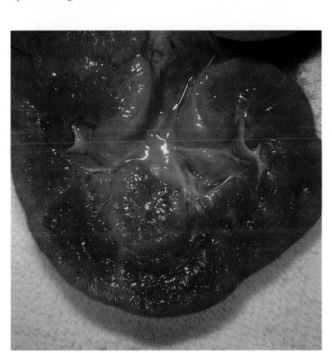

FIGURE 9–17. Sponge kidney

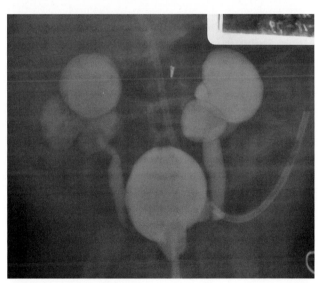

FIGURE 9–19. Hydronephrosis

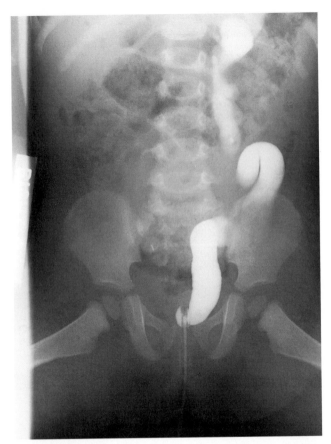

FIGURE 9–20. Hydroureter

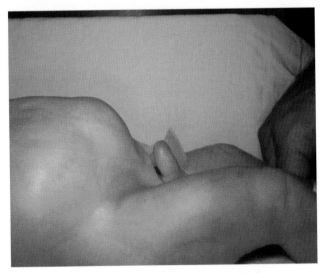

FIGURE 9–21. Distended bladder: posterior urethral valves

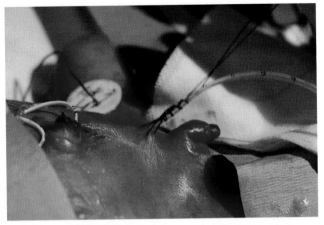

FIGURE 9–22. Suprapubic catheter to decompress a distended bladder

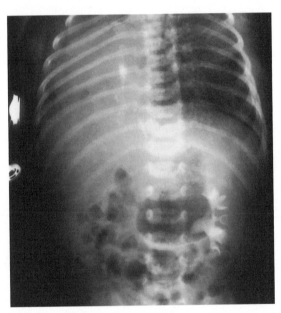

FIGURE 9–23. Thoracic ectopic kidney

EXSTROPHY

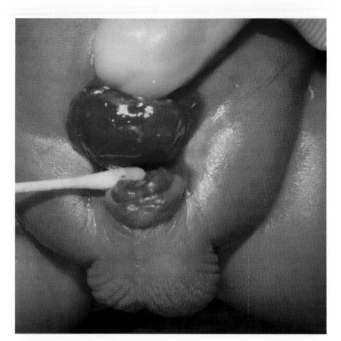

FIGURE 9–24. Bladder exstrophy, male

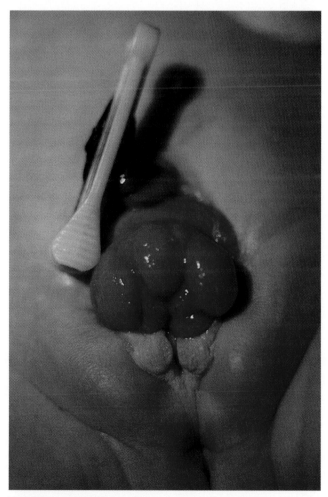

FIGURE 9–25. Bladder exstrophy, female—preoperative

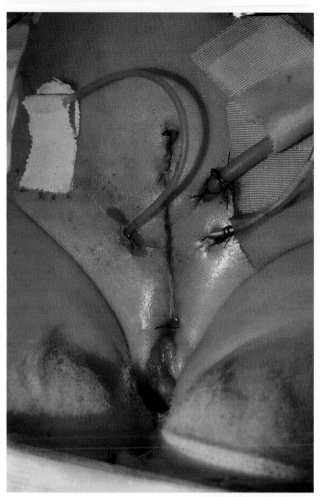

FIGURE 9–26. Bladder exstrophy, female—postoperative

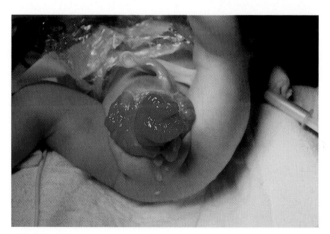

FIGURE 9–27. Cloacal exstrophy

URACHUS

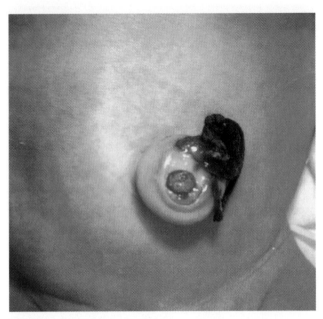

FIGURE 9–28. Patent urachus

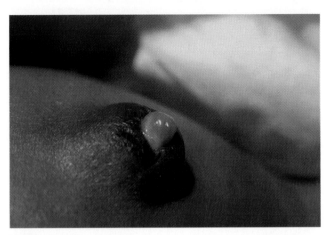

FIGURE 9–29. Urachal cyst

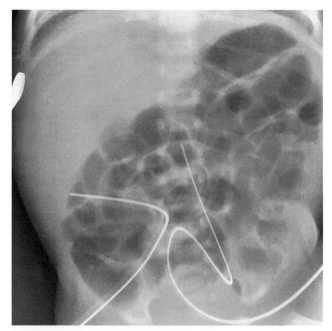

FIGURE 9–30. Omphalomesenteric remnant

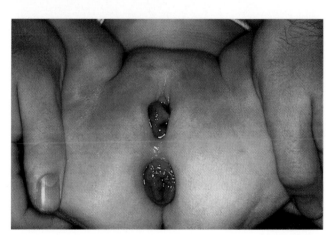

FIGURE 9–31. Ureterocele

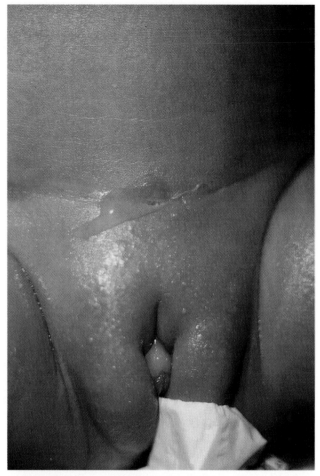

FIGURE 9–32. Cystocutaneous fistula

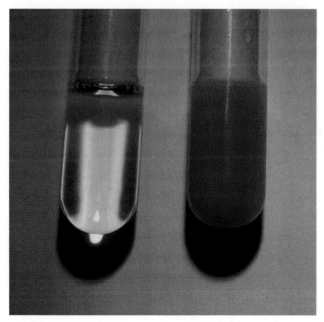

FIGURE 9–33. Crystalluria: calcium oxalate crystals in opaque urine (right)

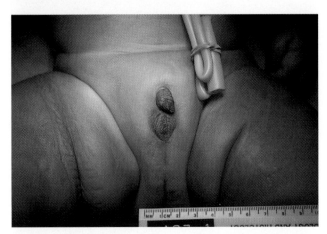

FIGURE 9–34. Micropenis: normal chromosomes, no metabolic defect detected

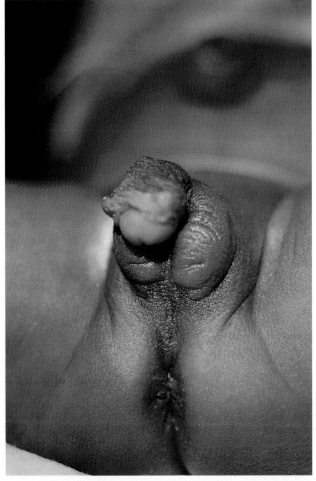

FIGURE 9–35. Hooded prepuce

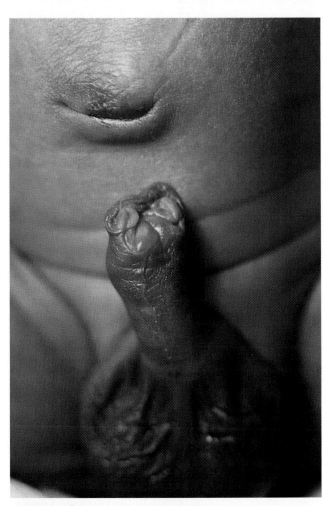

FIGURE 9–36. Hypospadias: Glans and shaft

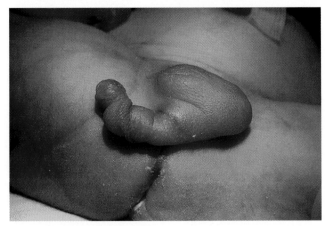

FIGURE 9–37. Anteverted penis

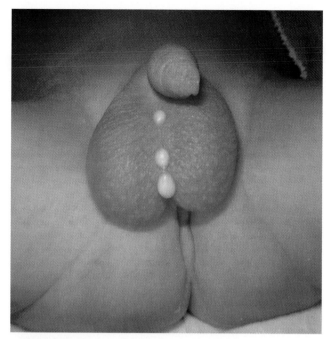

FIGURE 9–38. Inclusion cysts of median raphe

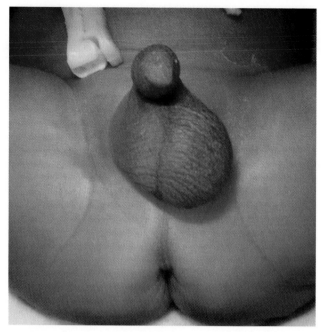

FIGURE 9–40. Right undescended testis

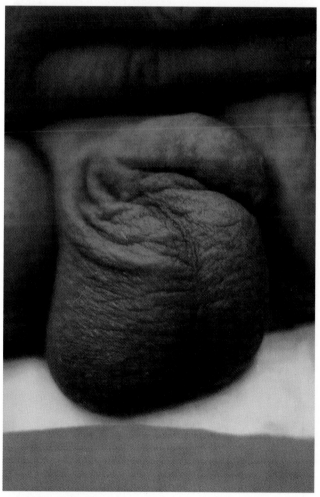

FIGURE 9–39. Bilateral hydrocele

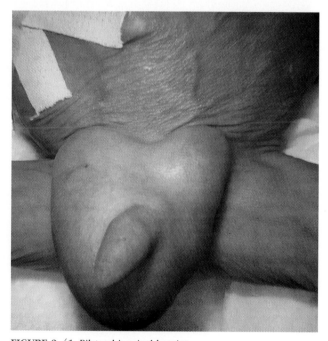

FIGURE 9–41. Bilateral inguinal hernias

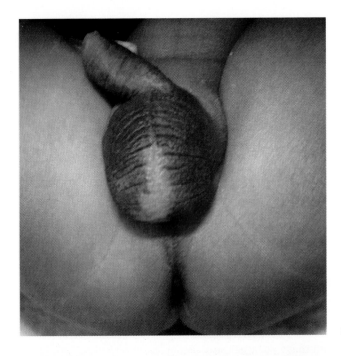

FIGURE 9–42. Scrotal vitiligo

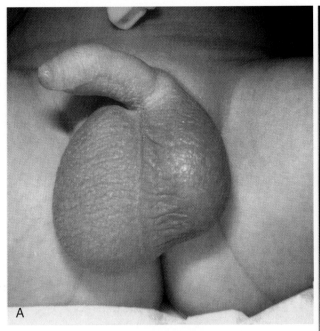

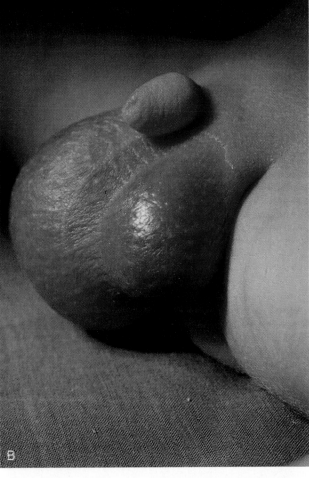

FIGURE 9–43. A and B, Testicular torsion

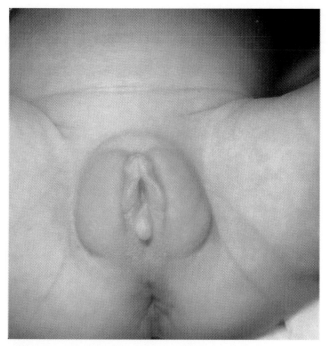

FIGURE 9-44. Vaginal tag

HYDROMETROCOLPOS

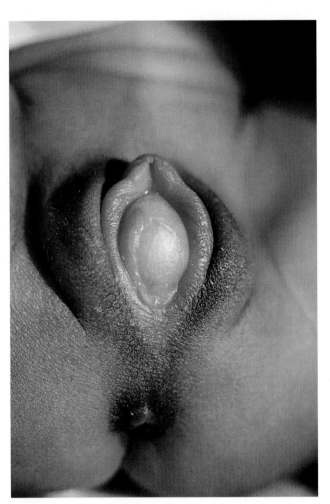

FIGURE 9–45. Intact hymen

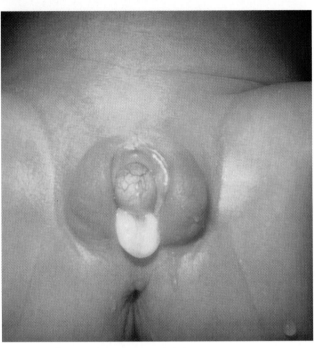

FIGURE 9–47. Cruciate incision and drainage

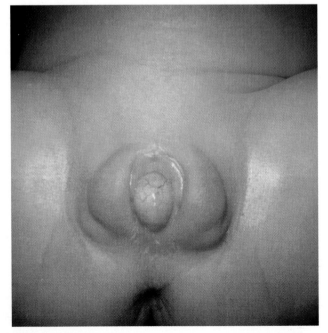

FIGURE 9–46. Intact hymen

SELECTED REFERENCES

Bailie MD, Ed. (1992) Renal Function and Disease. Clin Perinatol 19:1.

Jones KL. (1997) Smith's Recognizable Patterns of Human Malformation, 5th ed. Philadelphia, WB Saunders.

Kenner C and Brueggemeyer A. Assessment and management of genitourinary dysfunction. *In* Kenner C, Brueggemeyer A, and Gunderson LP, Eds. (1993) Comprehensive Neonatal Nursing. Philadelphia, WB Saunders.

Moore KL and Persaud TVN. (1993) The Developing Human, 5th ed. Philadelphia, WB Saunders.

Polin RA and Fox WW. (1998) Fetal and Neonatal Physiology, 2nd ed. Philadelphia, WB Saunders, Chapters 142-155.

Taeusch HW and Ballard RA. (1998) Avery's Diseases of the Newborn, 7th ed. Philadelphia, WB Saunders, Chapters 91-94.

10 Endocrine

The absence of an endocrine organ commonly delays the maturation and function of tissues dependent on the hormones produced by that gland. Genetically inherited enzyme defects in hormone metabolism result in endocrine disorders and abnormal sexual differentiation.

Table 10-1 gives an overview of the early fetal development of the endocrine organs. Maternal hormones may have an effect on the fetus. Placental hormones help maintain the pregnancy in early gestation. Some of the important common hormones, thyroid-stimulating hormone, insulin, and growth hormone, can be detected prior to 20 weeks' gestation.

Disorders of sexual differentiation may present in a very dramatic way as ambiguous genitalia. The two most common varieties are the incompletely masculinized

TABLE 10-1

DEVELOPMENT OF ENDOCRINE ORGANS	
Wks	
5.5	Adrenal cortex
7.5	Parathyroid
	Sympathetic neuroblasts
8	Thyroid follicles
10	Epinephrine, norepinephrine
11	Thyroid-stimulating hormone
12	Anterior pituitary—acidophilic granules
	Ovary—primitive follicles
	Testes—Leydig cells
	Insulin detected
16	Anterior pituitary—basophilic granules
18-20	Growth hormone
26-28	Testes descend
40+	Adrenal: regression of fetal zone

TABLE 10-2

PREVALENCE OF NEONATAL THYROID DISORDERS	
Thyroid dysgenesis	1:4000
Agenesis	
Ectopia	
Transient hypothyroidism	1:30,000
Prematurity	
Drug-induced	
Maternal antibody	
Thyroid dysmorphogenesis	1:30,000
Thyroglobulin defect	
Thyroid stimulating hormone (TSH) receptor defect	
Iodide-trapping defect	
Organification defect	
Iodotyrosine deiodinase defect	
Hypothalamus—pituitary defect	1:100,000
Panhypopituitarism	
Thyroid stimulating hormone deficiency	

46,XY male fetus and the inappropriate masculinization of the genitalia of a 46,XX fetus with ovaries. The latter usually results from androgen excess due to one of a number of different adrenal enzyme deficiencies, most commonly 21-hydroxylase deficiency. The majority of these enzyme deficiencies are inherited in an autosomal recessive manner. The incidence of all of forms of congenital adrenal hyperplasia is 1 in 500 to 1 in 5000 newborn infants.

Thyroid hormones are essential for development of many organs, especially the brain. Approximately 1 in 4000 newborn infants has congenital hypothyroidism. Thyroid dysgenesis is the most common, but other etiologies are noted in Table 10-2.

THYROID

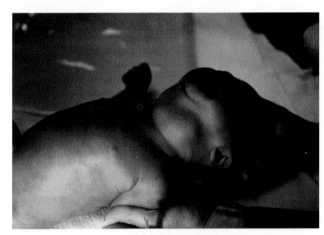

FIGURE 10–1. Goiter: maternal Graves disease

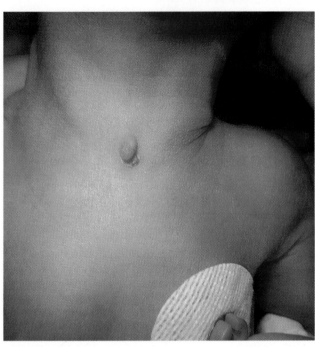

FIGURE 10–3. Ectopic thyroid

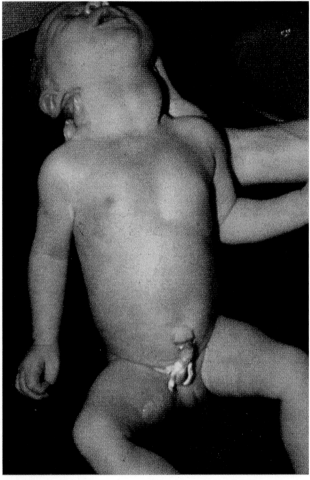

FIGURE 10–2. Goiter: iodine deficiency

HYPOPITUITARISM

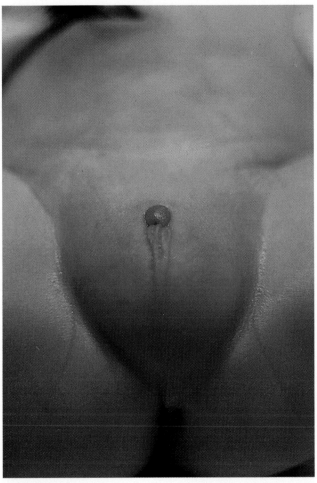

FIGURE 10–4. Micropenis

AMBIGUOUS GENITALIA

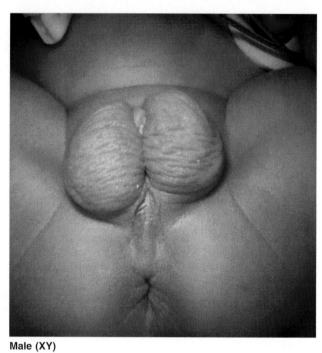

Male (XY)

FIGURE 10–5. Testes in labioscrotal folds—androgen insensitivity

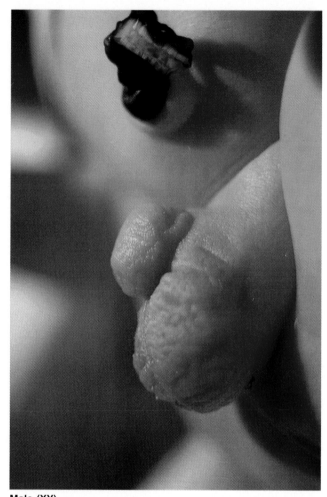

Male (XY)

FIGURE 10–6. Phallic segmentation

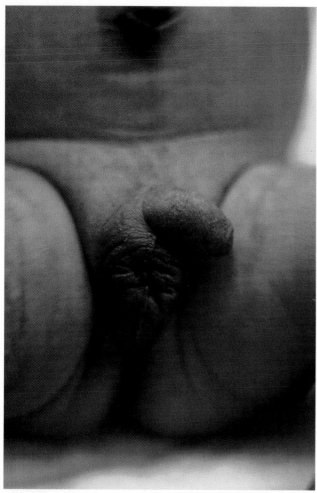

Male (XY)

FIGURE 10–7. Small phallus, undescended testes

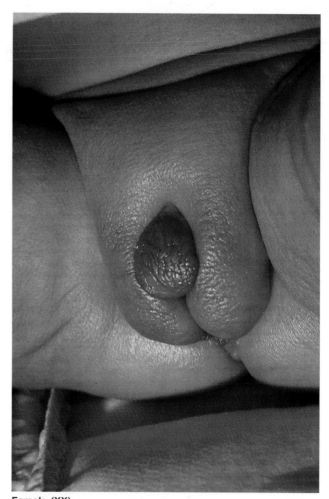

Female (XX)

FIGURE 10–8. Clitoral enlargement

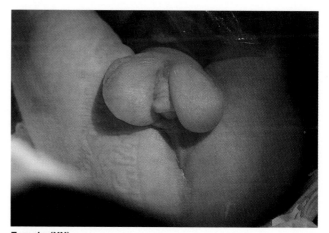

Female (XX)

FIGURE 10–9. Labial hypertrophy

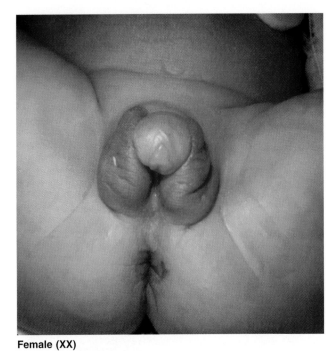

Female (XX)

FIGURE 10–10. 21-Hydroxylase deficiency

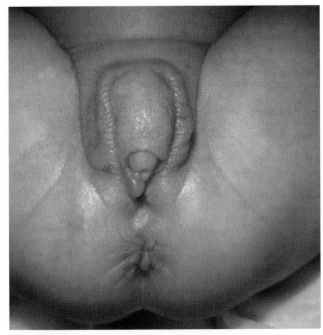

Female (XX)

FIGURE 10–11. 13-Hydroxylase deficiency

MATERNAL ESTROGEN EFFECT

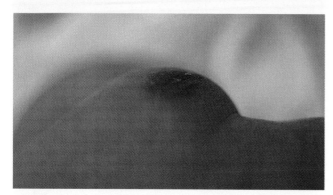

FIGURE 10–12. Breast hypertrophy

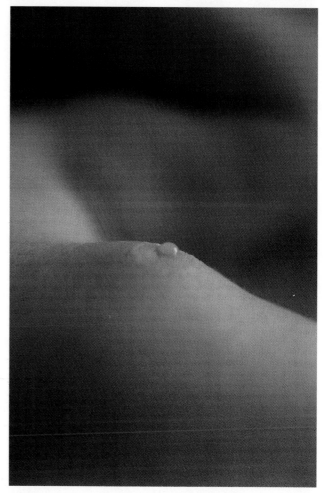

FIGURE 10–13. Witch's milk

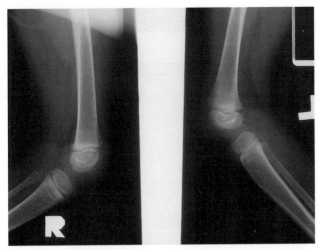

FIGURE 10–14. Rickets: decreased bone density, flared epiphyses

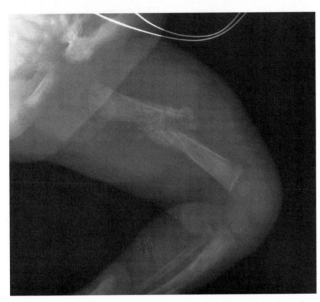

FIGURE 10–15. Osteopenia of prematurity: fractured femur in a 4 month old, 600-gm birthweight baby

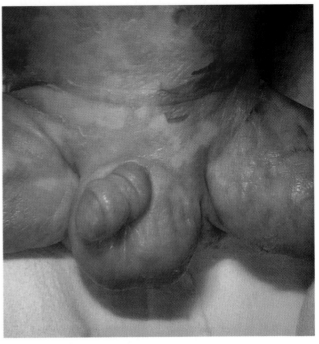

FIGURE 10–16. Essential fatty acid deficiency

SELECTED REFERENCES

Gamblien V et al. Assessment and management of endocrine dysfunction. *In* Kenner C, Brueggemeyer A, and Gunderson LP, Eds. (1993) Comprehensive Neonatal Nursing. Philadelphia, WB Saunders.

Jones KL. (1997) Smith's Recognizable Patterns of Human Malformation, 5th ed. Philadelphia, WB Saunders.

Moore KL and Persaud TVN. (1993) The Developing Human, 5th ed. Philadelphia, WB Saunders.

Polin RA and Fox WW. (1998) Fetal and Neonatal Physiology, 2nd ed. Philadelphia, WB Saunders, Chapters 222–228.

Taeusch HW and Ballard RA. (1998) Avery's Diseases of the Newborn, 7th ed. Philadelphia, WB Saunders, Chapters 100–102.

11 Musculoskeletal

The musculoskeletal system is divided into two major components. The axial skeletal system includes the cranium, vertebral column, ribs, and sternum, whereas the appendicular skeleton comprises the bones of the limbs. Table 11–1 gives an overview of the development of the musculoskeletal system. Since the axial skeleton forms in close proximity to the central nervous system and the major intrathoracic and abdominal organs, defects in its development are far more serious than those of limb deformities. These include serious problems such as neural tube defects with spinal dysraphism, lethal thoracic dystrophies, and severe skeletal dysplasias.

Limb defects are rarely life-threatening. The etiology of the majority of limb anomalies is multifactorial—that is, they result from an interaction of both genetic and environmental factors. With the exception of thalidomide, it is difficult to attribute congenital anomalies of the limbs to specific environmental teratogens.

Parallel with the development of the extremities is the development of the muscular system, which arises from embryonic myoblasts that are derived from mesoderm. The majority of skeletal muscles develop before birth, and most all the remaining muscles are formed by the end of the first year of life. Increase in muscle size results in the formation of more myofilaments, which results in increased diameter of the fibers. Muscles increase in length and width proportionate to skeletal growth.

A rare condition, arthrogryposis multiplex congenita, consists of failure of normal muscle development, which leads to immobility of multiple joints. Many other forms of muscular dystrophy do not present in the immediate newborn period but become obvious as the infant fails to achieve milestones, including sitting, crawling, and walking.

TABLE 11–1

DEVELOPMENT OF THE MUSCULOSKELETAL SYSTEM	
30 days	Arm bud
34 days	Leg bud
38 days	Hand plate; innervation
44 days	Finger rays
	Elbow
7 wks	Cartilage models of bones
	Tail regression
8 wks	Movement
	Early ossification of long bones and sternum
10 wks	Joints
16 wks	Distinct bones
38 wks	Epiphyseal centers

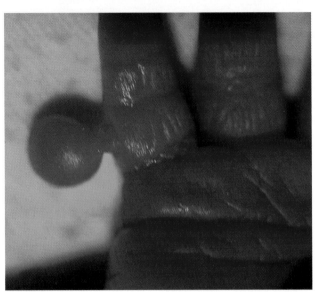

Accessory Digit

FIGURE 11–1. Stalked

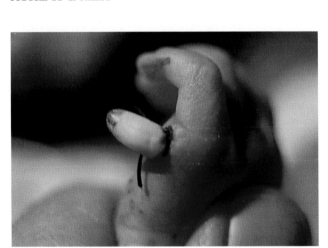

Accessory Digit

FIGURE 11–2. Ligated

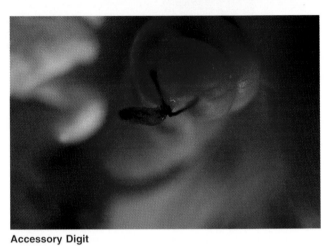

Accessory Digit

FIGURE 11–3. Dry necrosis

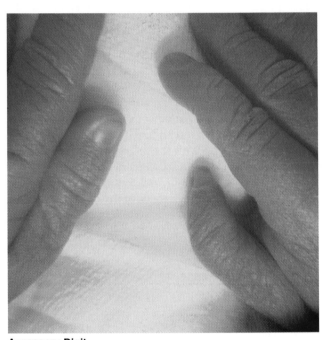

Accessory Digit

FIGURE 11–4. Thumb hypoplasia

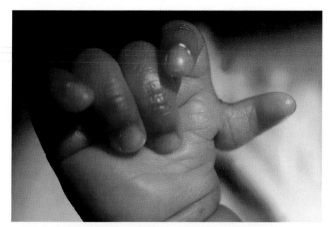

FIGURE 11–5. Disjointed thumb

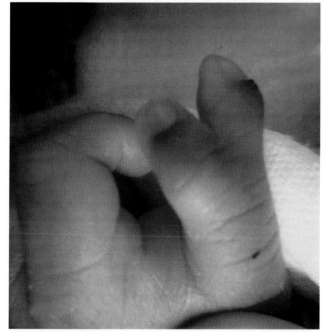

FIGURE 11–6. Bifid thumb

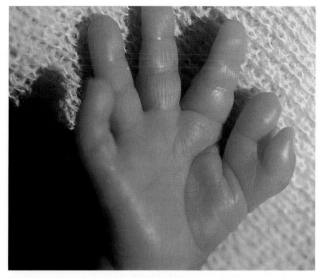

FIGURE 11–7. Hypoplastic bifid thumb

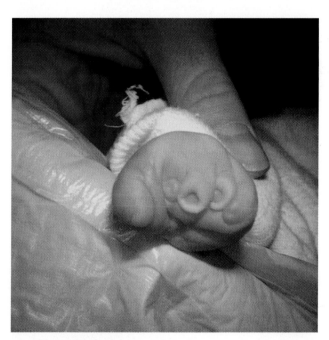

FIGURE 11–8. Hypoplastic hand with nails

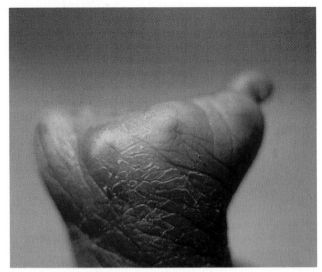

Aplastic Digits with Abnormal Thumb

FIGURE 11–9. Absent fingers, hypoplastic

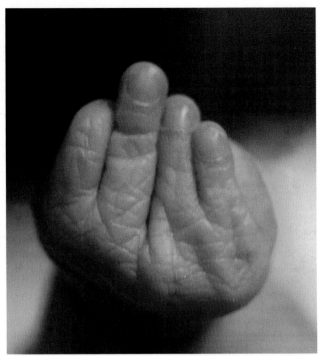

FIGURE 11–11. Shortened digits

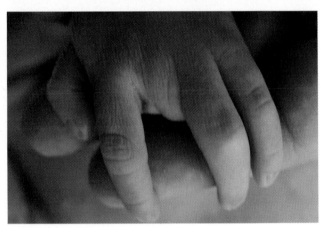

FIGURE 11–12. Absent middle finger

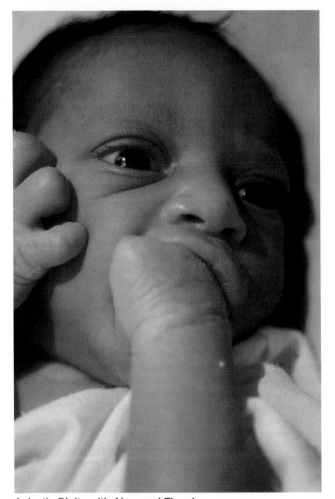

Aplastic Digits with Abnormal Thumb

FIGURE 11–10. Infant preferentially sucking the malformed hand

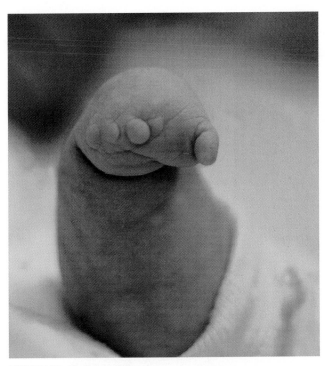

FIGURE 11–13. Palmar hypoplasia

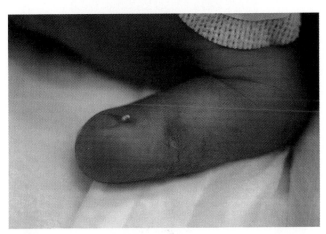

FIGURE 11–14. Absent hand

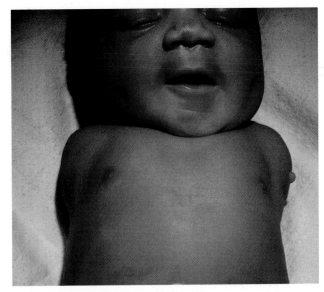

FIGURE 11–15. Amelia—anterior view

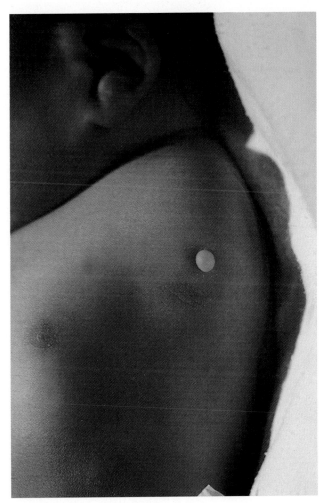

FIGURE 11–16. Amelia—lateral view

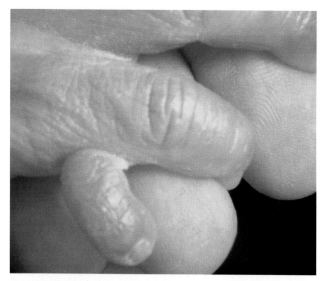

FIGURE 11–17. Polydactyly

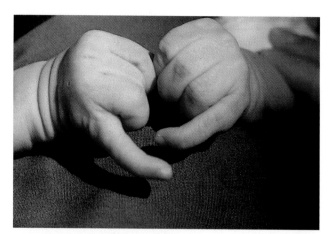

FIGURE 11–18. Elongated 5th fingers

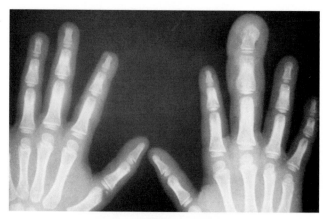

FIGURE 11–19. Radiograph of hypertrophic digit

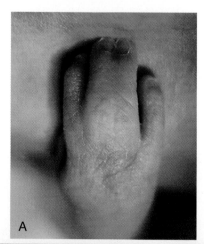

A

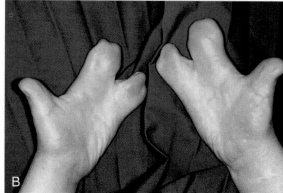

B

FIGURE 11–20 *A* and *B*. Two variations of syndactyly of fingers

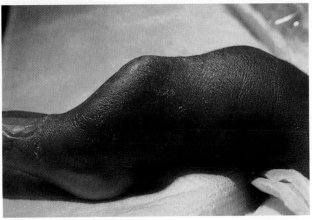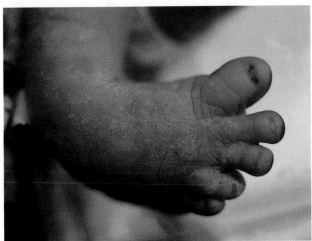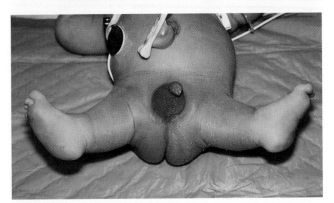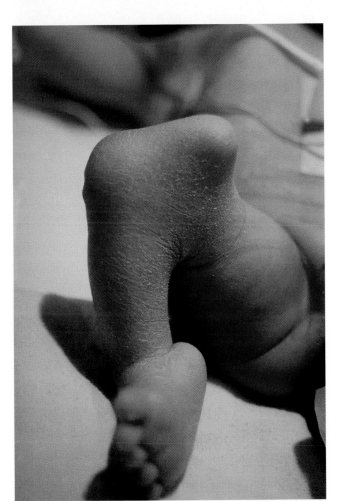

LOWER EXTREMITIES

FIGURE 11–21. Absent femurs

FIGURE 11–23. Deformed tibia

FIGURE 11–24. Clubfoot

FIGURE 11–22. Anomalous femur, hypoplastic tibia

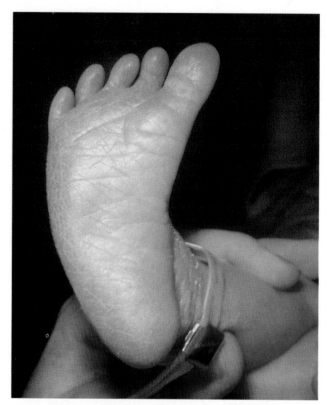

FIGURE 11–25. Metatarsus adductus

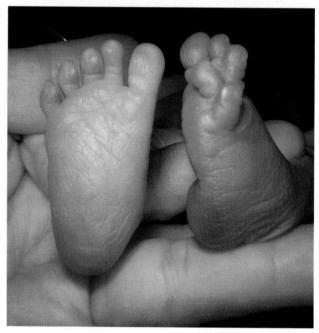

FIGURE 11–26. Oligohydramnios compressed foot

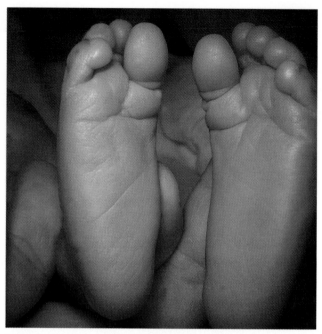

FIGURE 11–27. Ray deformity—midfoot hypoplasia

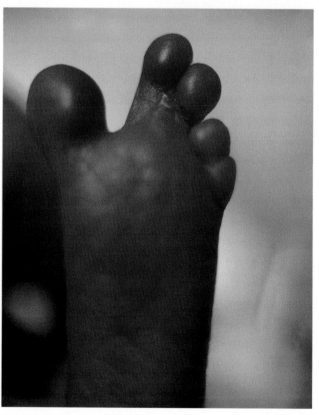

FIGURE 11–28. Toe syndactyly

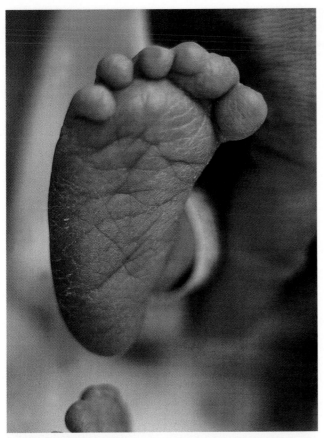

FIGURE 11–29. Polydactyly

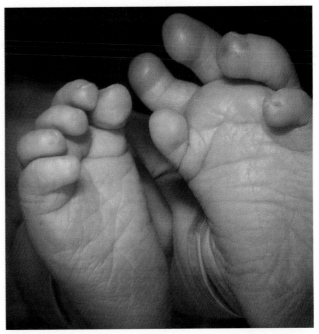

FIGURE 11–31. Hemihypertrophy of left foot

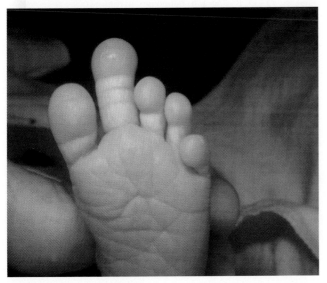

FIGURE 11–30. Macrodactyly

JEUNE SYNDROME

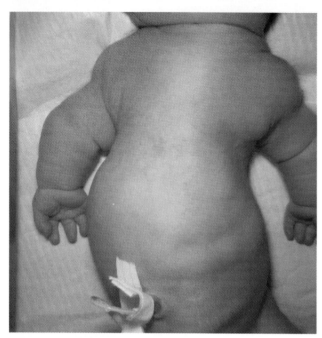

FIGURE 11–32. Thoracodystrophy

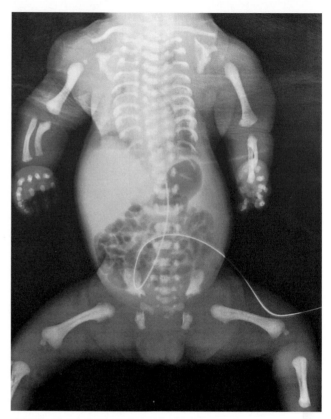

FIGURE 11–33. Radiograph: pulmonary hypoplasia

ACHONDROPLASTIC DWARF

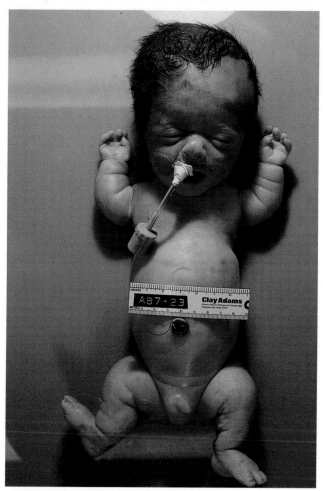

FIGURE 11–34. Small thorax, shortened limbs

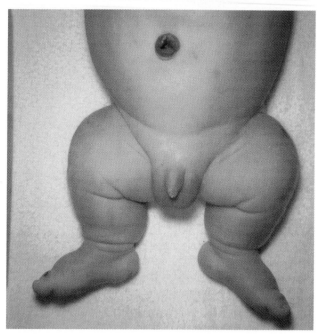

FIGURE 11–35. Short femurs and tibias

CAMPTOMELIC DWARF

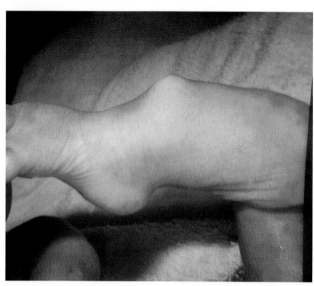

FIGURE 11–36. Bowed tibia

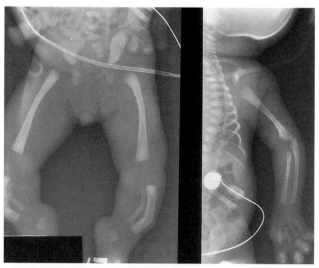

FIGURE 11–37. Radiograph: deformities of distal long bones

ARTHROGRYPOSIS

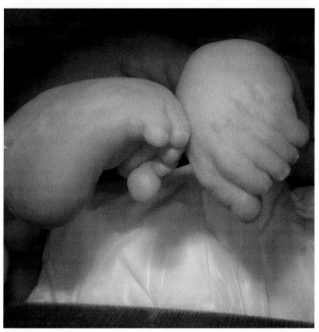

FIGURE 11–38. Feet

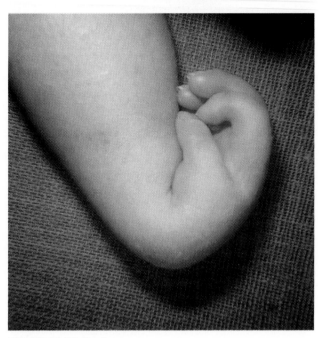

FIGURE 11–39. Hand

OSTEOGENESIS IMPERFECTA

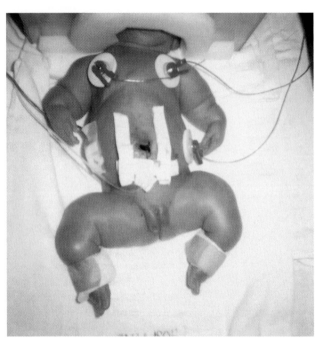

FIGURE 11–40. Swollen extremities from multiple fractures

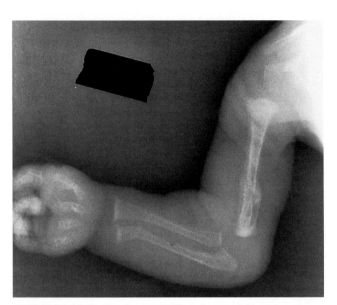

FIGURE 11–42. Healing fractures of long bones of the arm

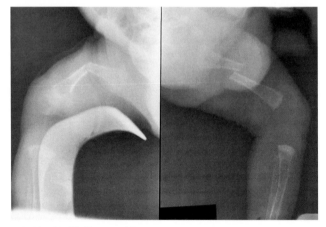

FIGURE 11–41. Fractured femurs

POLAND SYNDROME

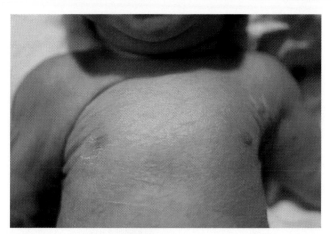

FIGURE 11–43. Poland syndrome

CAUDAL REGRESSION

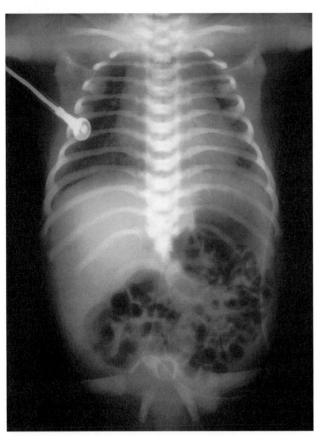

FIGURE 11–44. Absent lumbar spine

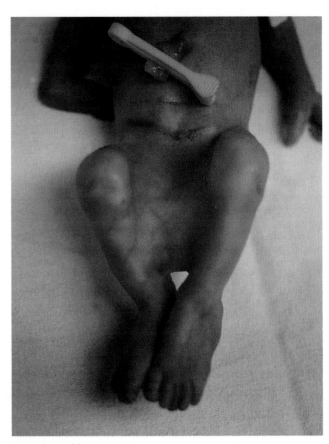

FIGURE 11–46. Webbed legs

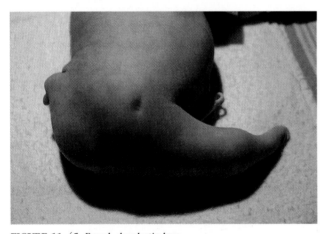

FIGURE 11–45. Fused, dysplastic legs

SELECTED REFERENCES

Butler J. Assessment and management of musculoskeletal dysfunction. *In* Kenner C, Brueggemeyer A, and Gunderson LP, Eds. (1993) Comprehensive Neonatal Nursing. Philadelphia, WB Saunders.

Jones KL. (1997) Smith's Recognizable Patterns of Human Malformation, 5th ed. Philadelphia, WB Saunders.

Moore KL and Persaud TVN. (1993) The Developing Human, 5th ed. Philadelphia, WB Saunders.

Polin RA and Fox WW. (1998) Fetal and Neonatal Physiology, 2nd ed. Philadelphia, WB Saunders, Chapters 208–215.

Taeusch HW and Ballard RA. (1998) Avery's Diseases of the Newborn, 7th ed. Philadelphia, WB Saunders, Chapters 27, 31.

12 Hematology—Neoplasia

The cellular elements of blood must constantly be produced since they have limited life spans. The first of these to form in utero are the red blood cells; they are found circulating in the primitive vessels as early as 19 days of gestation. Table 12-1 provides an overview of the development of the hematopoietic elements.

During hematopoiesis development, multipotent stem cells, originally in the yolk sac and liver and then in the bone marrow, divide and differentiate to give the array of cellular components, each having its unique function and life span.

Although the typical red blood cell in the adult circulates for approximately 120 days, the life span of the larger red cell of the neonate is less than 100 days and in the preterm infant under metabolic stress may be as short as 60 days. Newborn infants have larger platelets, with a life span of approximately 7 to 8 days compared with 10 days for an adult. The circulating granulocytes (neutrophils and eosinophils) survive for less than 12 hours after release from the bone marrow.

Only thrombocytopenia, anemia, and polycythemia are easy to demonstrate in the neonate. Both thrombocytopenia and anemia result from either insufficient production or excess destruction of platelets or red blood cells. Beyond that generalization, a myriad of diseases cause thrombocytopenia or anemia.

Congenital tumors are rare and may affect any organ system. Since they are formed in the rapidly developing fetus, they commonly have primitive embryonic components and a high potential for malignancy.

TABLE 12-1

DEVELOPMENT OF HEMATOPOIESIS	
2-6 wks	Megaloblastic period (peak, 4 wks)
	Hemocytoblasts, derived from endothelial cells (angioblasts) of blood vessels in embryo and yolk sac
	Embryonic hemoglobins
	Gower I, Gower II, Portland
6-26 wks	Hepatic period (peak, 12 wks)
6 wks	Platelet precursors in fetal liver
8-12 wks	Most clotting factors and inhibitors
10 wks	Hemoglobin F
	Nucleated red blood cells
15 wks-term+	Myeloid period (peak, 24+ wks)
17 wks	Mature red blood cells
	Leukocytes formed in bone marrow of clavicle
18-20 wks	Stem cells differentiate to form T and B lymphocytes
26-34 wks	Rapid increase in granulocytes
Term	Hemoglobin F, 75%; A, 25%

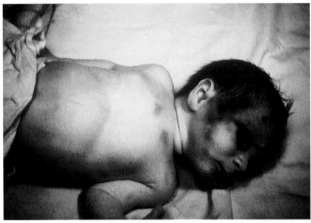

FIGURE 12–1. Thrombocytopenia due to immune-mediated platelet destruction

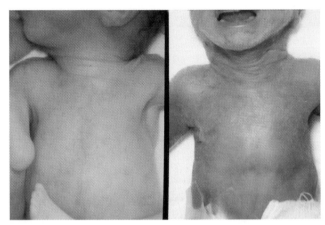

FIGURE 12–4. Twin (to placenta) to twin transfusion in identical preterm twins

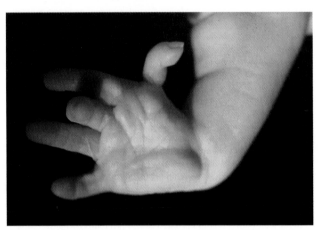

FIGURE 12–2. Thrombocytopenia: absent radius syndrome

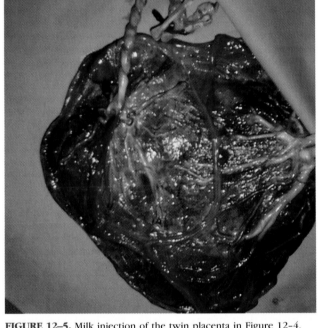

FIGURE 12–5. Milk injection of the twin placenta in Figure 12–4, showing connecting vessels

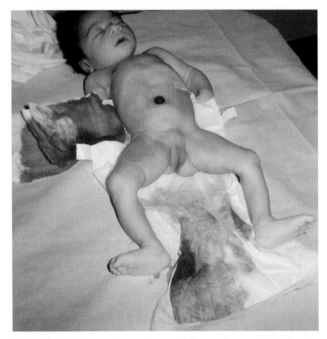

FIGURE 12–3. Hemorrhagic disease of the newborn: umbilical vein blood loss via the unclamped umbilical cord on the third day of life

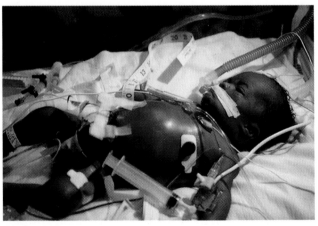

FIGURE 12–6. Hydrops fetalis due to severe Rh incompatibility

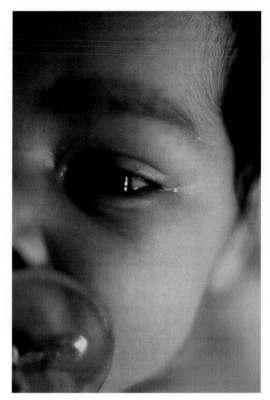

FIGURE 12–7. Jaundice due to congenital spherocytosis

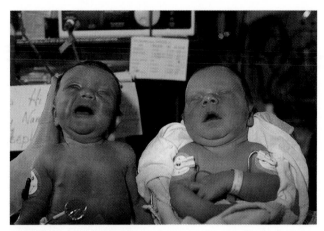

FIGURE 12–8. Bronzing of a baby (left) who had a high direct bilirubin fraction and received phototherapy

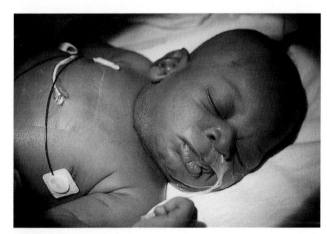

FIGURE 12–9. Jaundice due to tyrosinemia and hepatic dysfunction

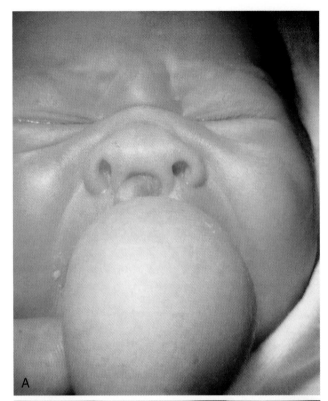

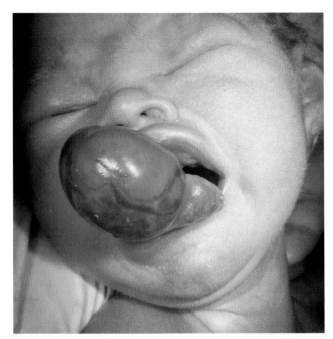

FIGURE 12–11. Hamartoma of the palate

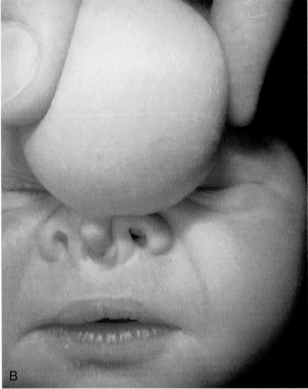

FIGURE 12–10. Dermoid of nasal septum. Two views demonstrating the mass (A) and stalk (B)

EPENDYMOMA

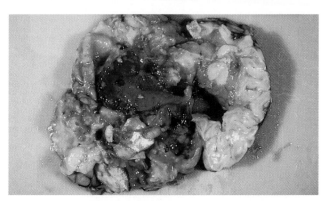

FIGURE 12–12. Gross pathology

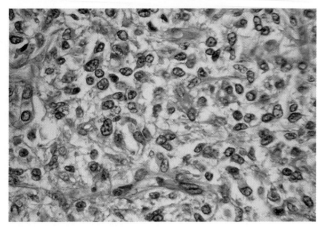

FIGURE 12–13. Microscopic pathology: rosettes, fibrils

NEUROECTODERMAL TUMOR—METASTATIC

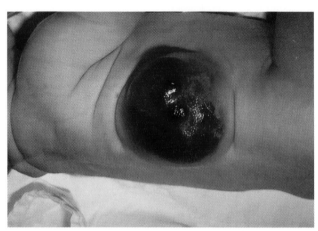

FIGURE 12–14. Back

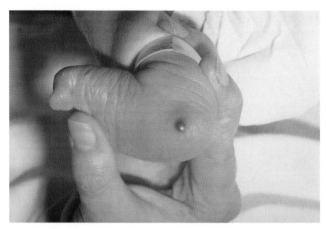

FIGURE 12–16. Foot

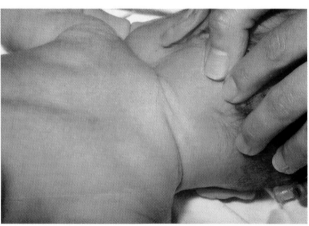

FIGURE 12–15. Neck

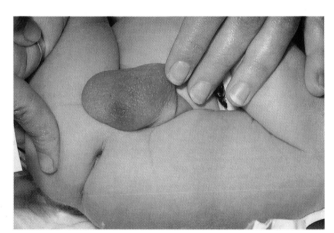

FIGURE 12–17. Scrotum

CYSTIC HYGROMA

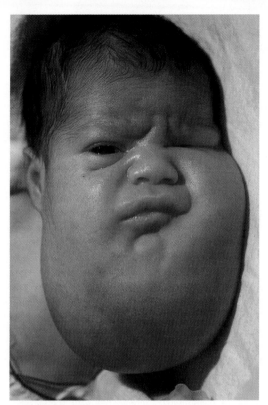

FIGURE 12–18. Face

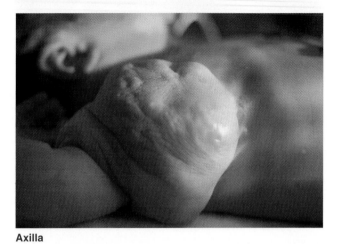

Axilla

FIGURE 12–20. Continued growth, 2 weeks later

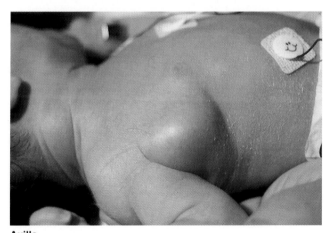

Axilla

FIGURE 12–19. At birth

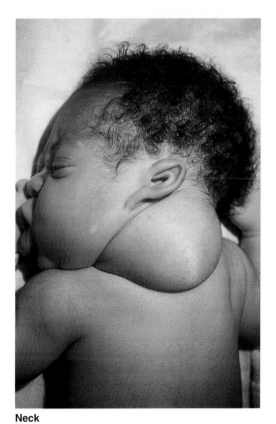

Neck

FIGURE 12–21. External appearance

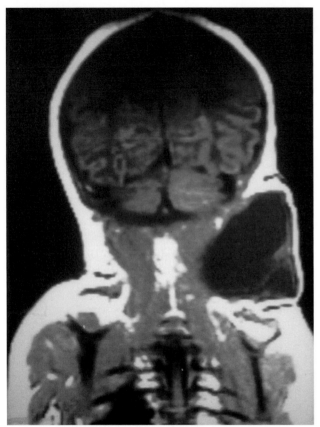

Neck

FIGURE 12–22. Computerized tomography scan, coronal

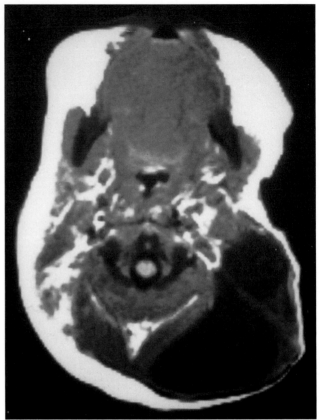

Neck

FIGURE 12–23. Computerized tomography scan, transverse

MESENCHYMOMA: CHEST WALL

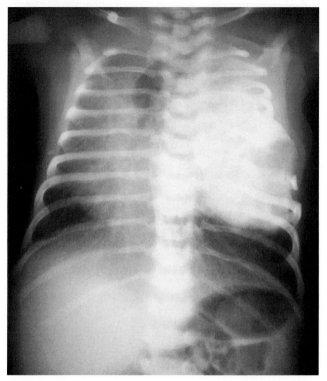

FIGURE 12–24. At birth

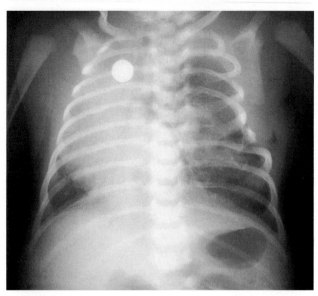

FIGURE 12–26. Postoperative

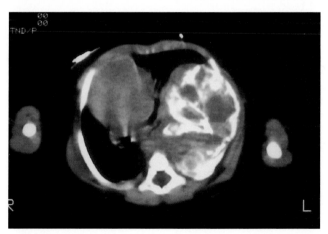

FIGURE 12–25. Computerized tomography scan

NEUROBLASTOMA

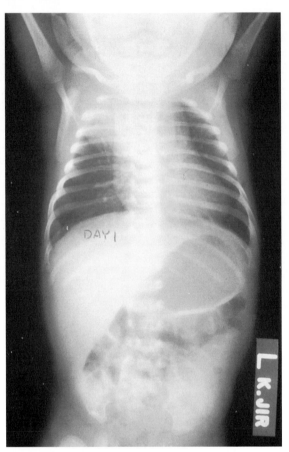

FIGURE 12–27. Radiograph: right upper chest

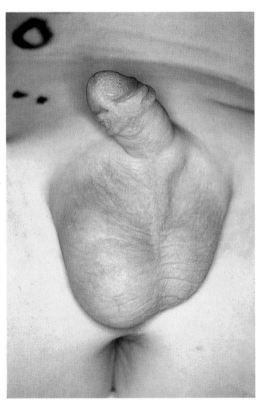

FIGURE 12–29. Metastatic to testis

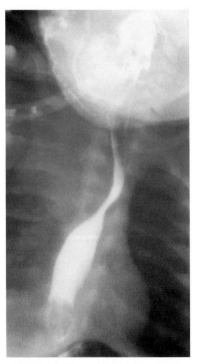

FIGURE 12–28. Barium swallow: impinging on esophagus

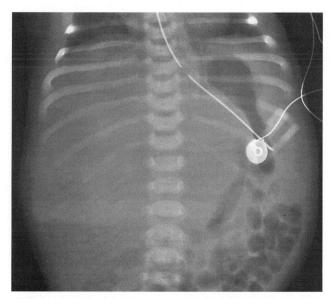

FIGURE 12–30. Radiograph: hepatic tumor calcification

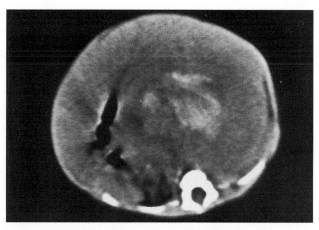

FIGURE 12–31. Computerized tomography scan: intrahepatic calcification

TUMOR

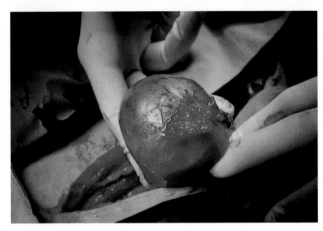

FIGURE 12–32. Ovarian tumor

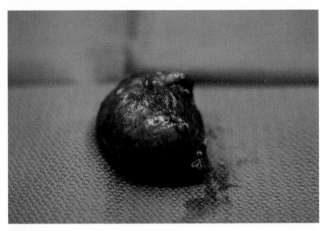

FIGURE 12–33. Adrenal tumor

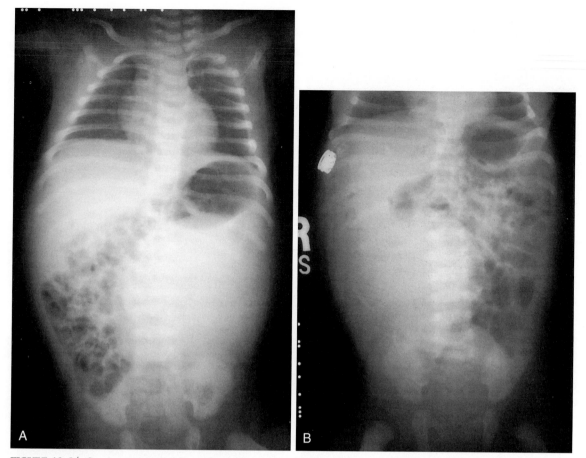

FIGURE 12–34. Ovarian cyst: two radiographs demonstrating shifting of the mass in the abdominal cavity

SACROCOCCYGEAL TERATOMA

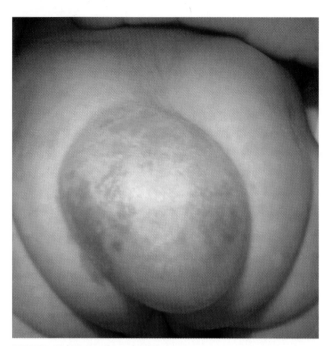

FIGURE 12–35. Small, no neural elements

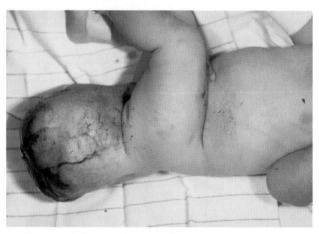

FIGURE 12–36. Large, with neural elements

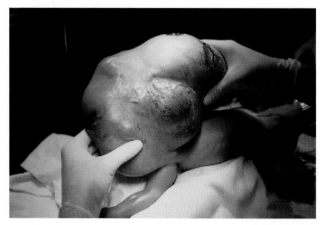

FIGURE 12–37. Massive sacrococcygeal teratoma comprising one quarter of the body weight

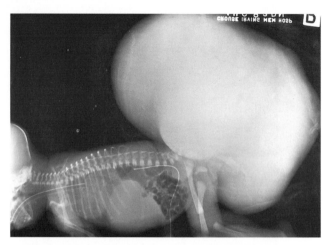

FIGURE 12–38. Radiograph: homogeneous density

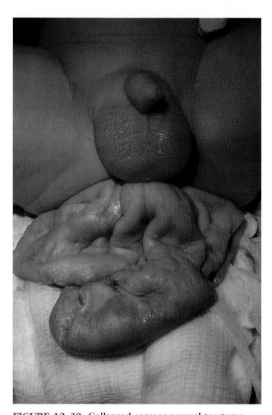

FIGURE 12–39. Collapsed sacrococcygeal teratoma

FIBROMA

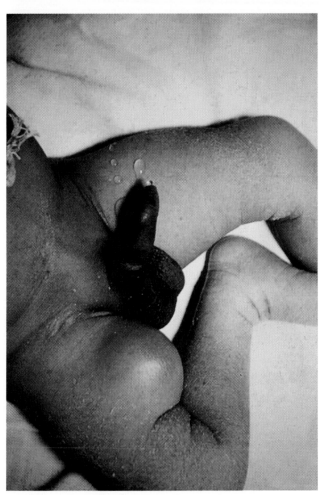

FIGURE 12–40. Fibroma of the thigh

SELECTED REFERENCES

Jones KL. (1997) Smith's Recognizable Patterns of Human Malformation, 5th ed. Philadelphia, WB Saunders.

Moore KL and Persaud TVN. (1993) The Developing Human, 5th ed. Philadelphia, WB Saunders.

Polin RA and Fox WW. (1998) Fetal and Neonatal Physiology, 2nd ed. Philadelphia, WB Saunders, Chapters 166–169.

Shawn N. Assessment and management of hematologic dysfunction. *In* Kenner C, Brueggemeyer A, and Gunderson LP, Eds. (1993) Comprehensive Neonatal Nursing. Philadelphia, WB Saunders.

Taeusch HW and Ballard RA. (1998) Avery's Diseases of the Newborn, 7th ed. Philadelphia, WB Saunders, Chapters 88–90.

Zipursky A. (1984) Pediatric Hematology. Clin Perinatol 11:2.

13 Dermatology

The skin of a newborn infant is a complex organ derived embryologically from both ectoderm and mesoderm. These contribute to the two distinct structural components, the epidermis and dermis, each with several elements. Embryologically, the ectoderm forms the epidermis, neural components, nails and hair, and sebaceous, apocrine, and sweat glands. The mesoderm contributes the dermal elements and associated subcutaneous fat and muscle. The chronology of fetal skin development is summarized briefly in Table 13–1.

The fetal periderm acts as a temporary barrier to the changing composition of amniotic fluid. It also serves as an active transport membrane between the embryo and its environment. At 12 to 16 weeks, the epidermis has an accumulation of glycogen, which is virtually absent by 34 weeks' gestation. However, there is significant regional variation in the newborn skin in thickness of the epidermis, control of subcutaneous blood flow, pigmentation, permeability, and surface chemistry.

Table 13–2 delineates the cutaneous structural differences between a preterm and a term infant. The skin of a term infant is very similar to that of an adult, with the greatest differences being the degree of pigmentation and ability to perspire. The skin of a preterm infant is more permeable with decreasing gestational age. A number of compounds have been identified that may produce metabolic acidosis, neurotoxicity, or structural damage. These include the iodine-containing soaps, aniline dyes, hexachlorophene, alpha-benzene hexachloride, and phenols.

The physiologic role of the skin is to provide barrier function, primarily at the level of the stratum corneum. The components of the physical barrier include mechanical, thermal, electromagnetic, chemical, and microbial barrier functions. The skin is also important in heat regulation and is much more efficient in the term infant than in the preterm infant. The preterm infant has difficulty maintaining temperature because of the decreased subcutaneous fat and the large surface area to mass ratio compared with that of a full-term infant. In addition, the nerve components are better developed in the term infant, who has a better perception of environmental stimuli than the preterm infant. The immunologic role of the skin in term and preterm babies has not been well characterized.

Biochemically, the pH of the skin is approximately 7.4 at birth. In the term infant, the pH decreases to 4.5 to 5.5 by the fifth day of life. This provides a bacteriostatic function for common cutaneous organisms. Concurrently, the ability of the skin to absorb ultraviolet radiation promoting the conversion of the ergosterol to vitamin D matures postnatally.

The sweat glands of a term infant are much better developed, so that by approximately 1 week after birth, salt and water excretion via sweat has matured. In the low birth weight infant the process takes much longer to develop. However, the infant born prematurely will have accelerated development of the sweat glands compared with the fetus.

TABLE 13–1

SKIN DEVELOPMENT OF THE FETUS	
WKS OF GESTATION	CHARACTERISTIC
3	Epidermis—single cell layer
5	Nerve tissue in dermis
6	Periderm appears
7	Mammary gland forms
8	Basal cell layer develops
10	Hair follicles and melanocytes appear
11	Dermis—collagen and elastic fibers
	Fingerprints
12	Fingernails, toenails, scalp and body hair appear
	Sebaceous glands
16	Sweat glands evident
17–19	Keratinization
	Migration of melanocytes to epidermal–dermal junction
	Dermal melanin produced
21–25	Skin translucent, capillaries visible
26–28	Subcutaneous fat
	Eccrine sweat glands mature but not fully functional
30–34	Prominent lanugo
	Fingernails reach tips of fingers
35–38	Toenails reach tips of toes

TABLE 13-2

STRUCTURAL COMPARISON OF THE SKIN OF PRETERM AND TERM NEONATES

STRUCTURE/FUNCTION	PRETERM (30 WKS)	TERM
Full-skin thickness	0.9 mm	1.2 m
Epidermal thickness	35-50 μ	50-60 μ
Stratum corneum thickness	4-5 μ	9-10 μ
	5 cell layers	15+ cell layers
Keratin filaments	Small bundles	Equal to adult
Collagen	Loosely organized	Smaller bundles than in adults
Melanosomes	1/3 of term	Equal to adult
Eccrine sweat glands	Reduced sweating	Reduced sweating
	13-24 days	2-5 days
Permeability	High	Effective barrier

The skin of a neonate reflects systemic illness, e.g., jaundice, cyanosis, plethora. Nutritional problems, such as essential fatty acid or zinc deficiency, have a characteristic scaling skin. Many transplacental congenital infections have cutaneous manifestations.

The following photographs provide an overview of the major neonatal dermatology findings.

WAARDENBURG SYNDROME

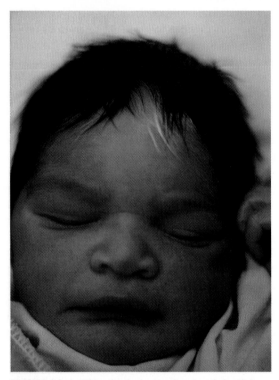

FIGURE 13–1. White forelock, associated with familial deafness (Waardenburg syndrome)

CUTIS APLASIA

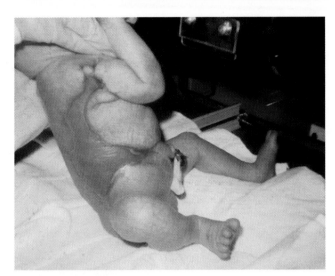

FIGURE 13–2. Trunk

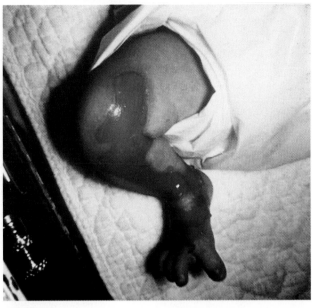

FIGURE 13–4. Leg

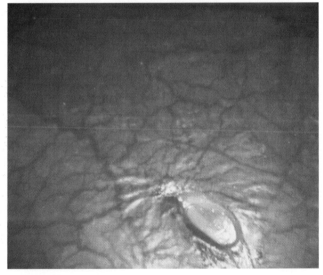

FIGURE 13–3. Scalp

ALBINO

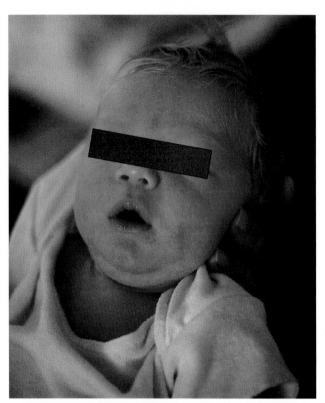

FIGURE 13–5. Caucasian neonate

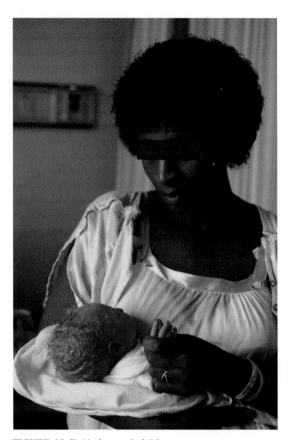

FIGURE 13–7. Mother and child

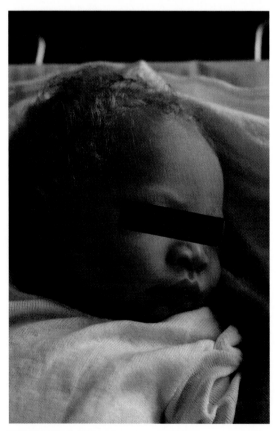

FIGURE 13–6. African-American neonate

PIEBALD/VITILIGO

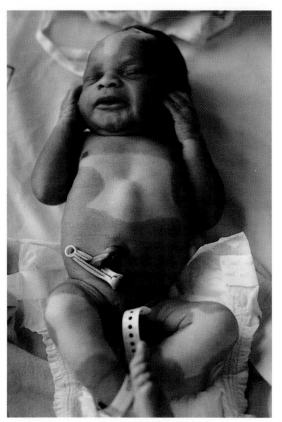

FIGURE 13–8. Trunk

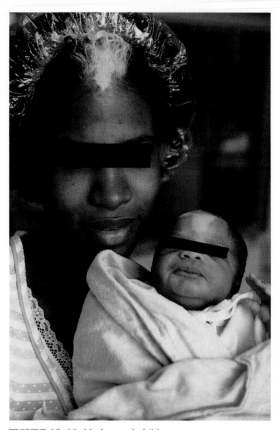

FIGURE 13–10. Mother and child

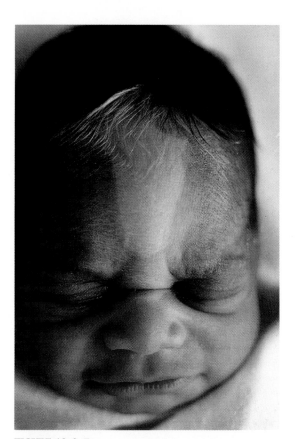

FIGURE 13–9. Face

CUTIS LAXA

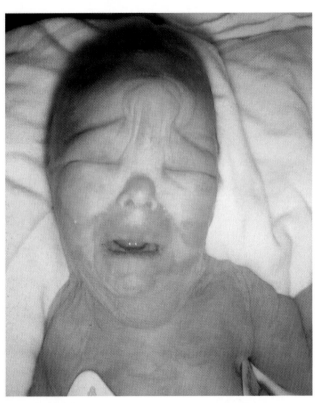

FIGURE 13–11. Face

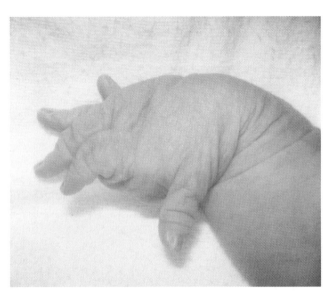

FIGURE 13–12. Hand

CONNECTIVE TISSUE DISORDER

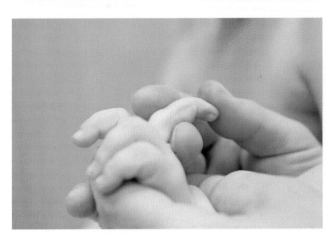

FIGURE 13–13. Ehlers-Danlos syndrome—finger

ICHTHYOSIS

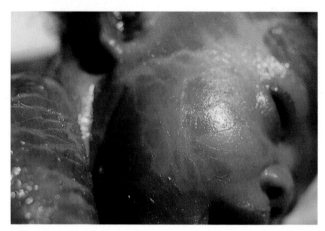

FIGURE 13–14. Face

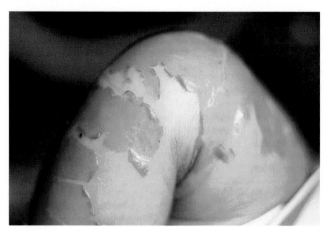

FIGURE 13–15. Extremity

HARLEQUIN

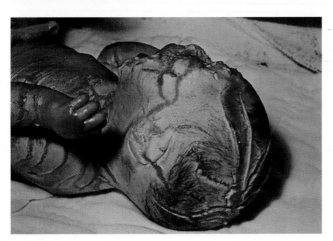

FIGURE 13–16. Scalp

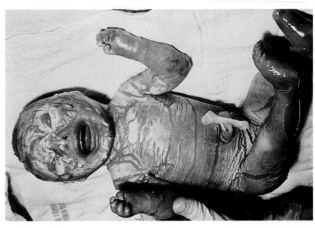

FIGURE 13–17. Trunk

EPIDERMOLYSIS BULLOSA

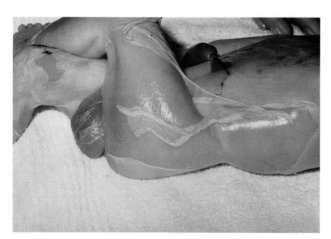

FIGURE 13–18. Trunk

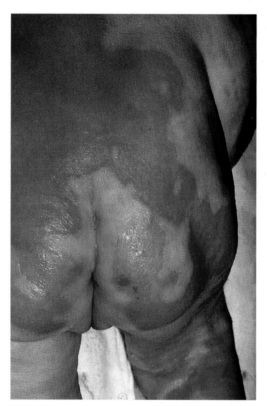

FIGURE 13–19. Back

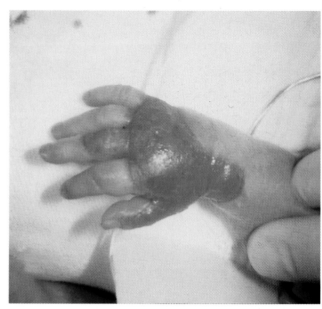

FIGURE 13–20. Hand

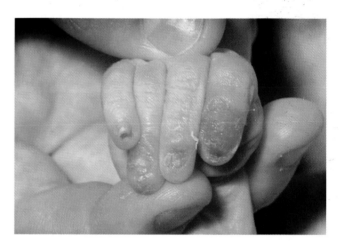

FIGURE 13–21. Fingers

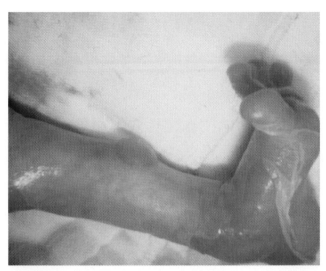

FIGURE 13–22. Foot

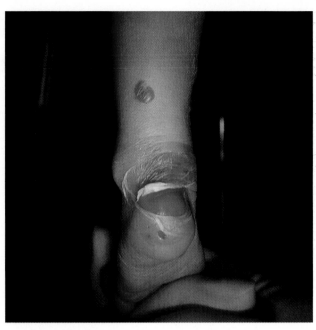

FIGURE 13–23. Heel

MILIARIA RUBRA

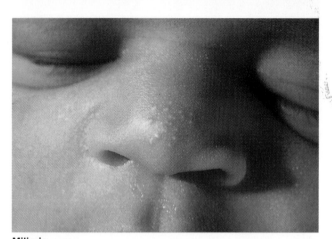

Miliaria

FIGURE 13–24. Nose

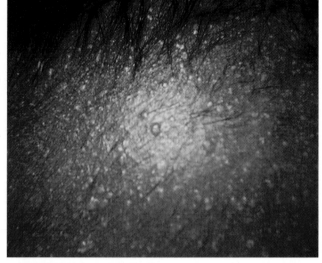

FIGURE 13–26. Miliaria crystallina

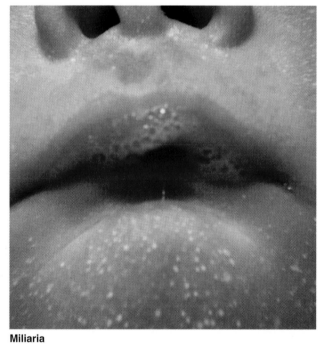

Miliaria

FIGURE 13–25. Face

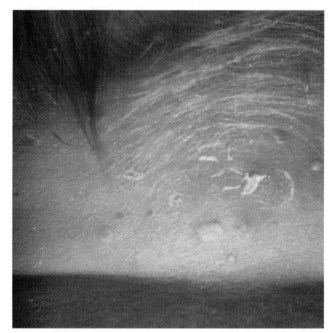

FIGURE 13–27. Miliaria pustulosa

MELANOSIS

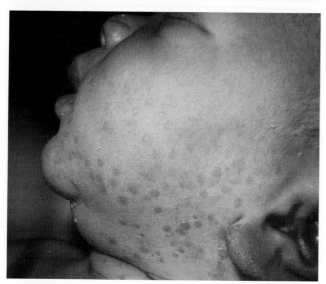

FIGURE 13–28. Pustular melanosis

ERYTHEMA

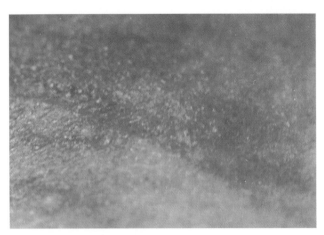

FIGURE 13–29. Erythema toxicum

FIGURE 13–30. Erythema multiforme

NEVUS FLAMMEUS—CAPILLARY HEMANGIOMA

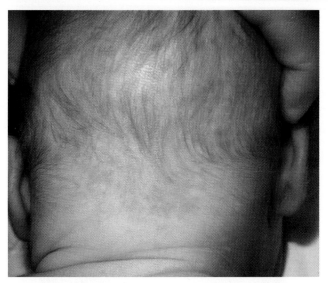

FIGURE 13–31. Neck

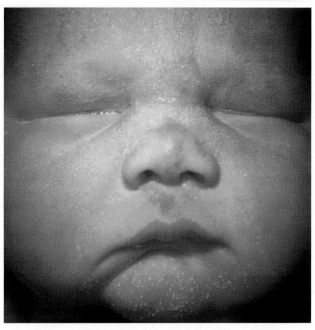

FIGURE 13–32. Face

FLAT HEMANGIOMA

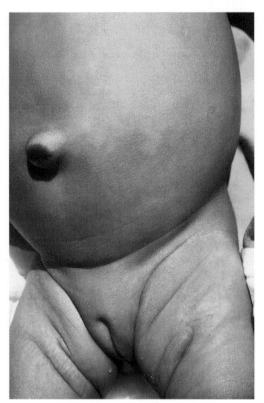

FIGURE 13–33. Groin

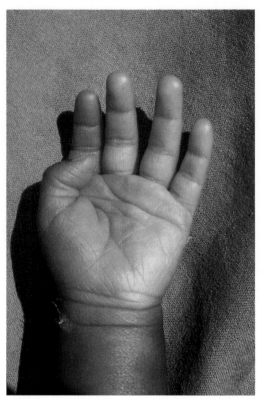

FIGURE 13–34. Hand

STRAWBERRY HEMANGIOMA

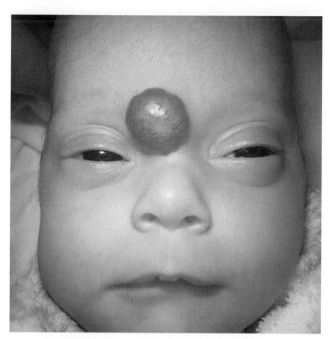

FIGURE 13–35. Forehead

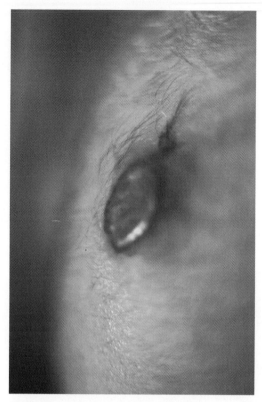

FIGURE 13–37. Early involution—flattened

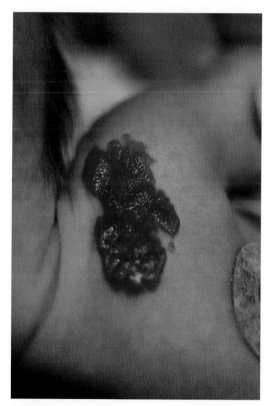

FIGURE 13–36. Shoulder

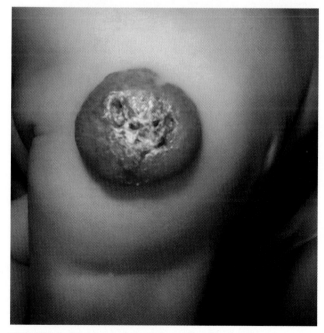

FIGURE 13–38. Advanced involution with central sealing

CAVERNOUS HEMANGIOMA

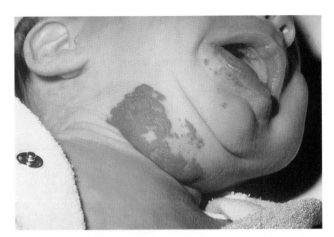

FIGURE 13–39. Neck

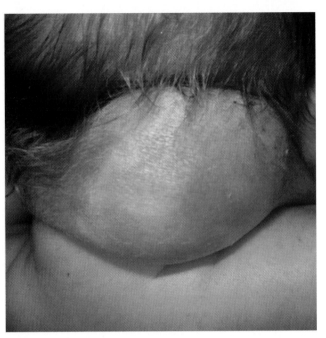

FIGURE 13–41. Neck

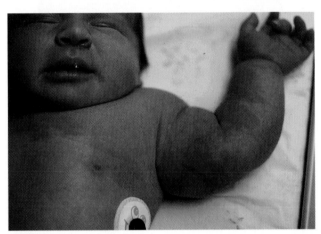

FIGURE 13–40. Shoulder/arm

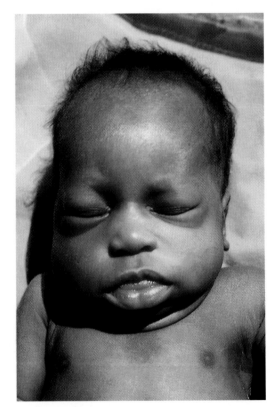

FIGURE 13–42. Face

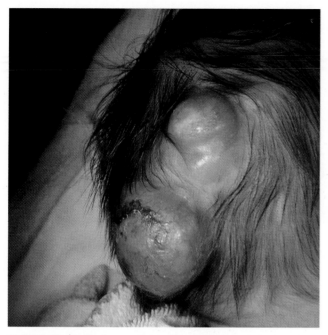

FIGURE 13–43. Lipohemangioma of the scalp

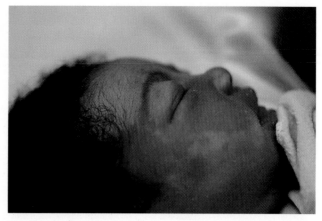

FIGURE 13–45. Port wine stain

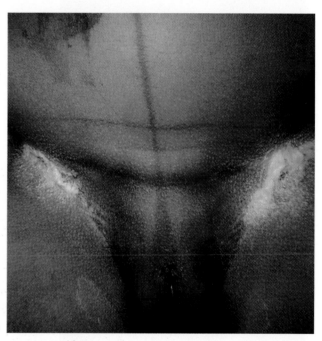

FIGURE 13–46. Linea nigra

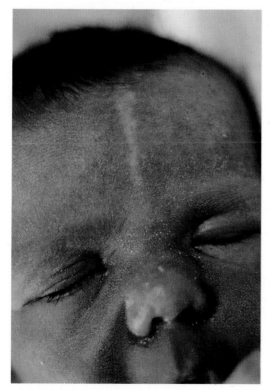

FIGURE 13–44. Sturge-Weber syndrome

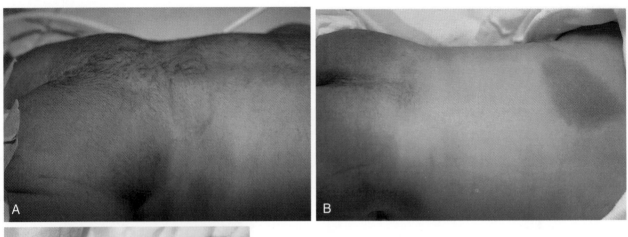

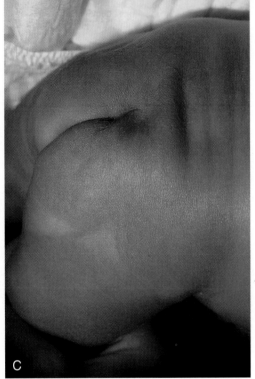

FIGURE 13–47. Mongolian spots (*A-C*)

NEVUS

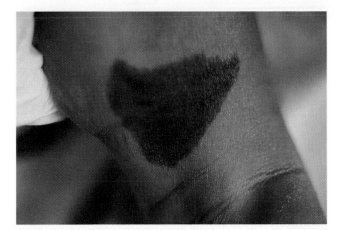

FIGURE 13–48. Leg, discrete margin

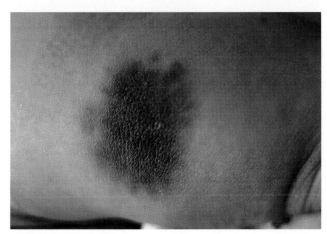

FIGURE 13–49. Diffuse margin

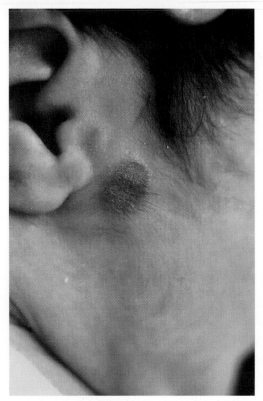

FIGURE 13–50. Preauricular

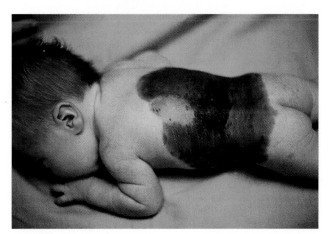

FIGURE 13–51. Bathing trunk

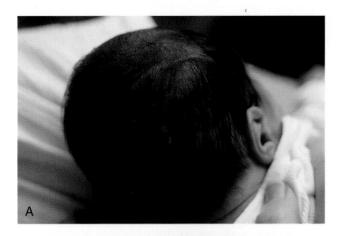

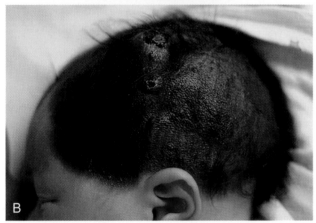

FIGURE 13–52. *A*, Scalp obscured by dark hair. *B*, Scalp.

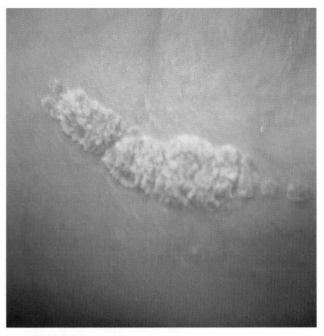

FIGURE 13–53. Nevus sebaceus

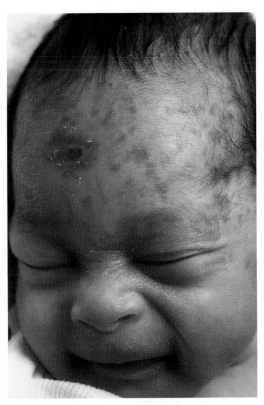

FIGURE 13–54. Neonatal lupus: a diffuse, purpuric, nodular rash

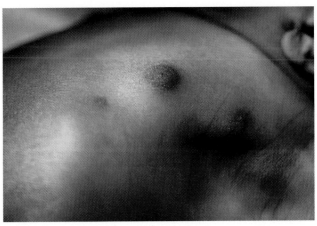

FIGURE 13–55. Accessory nipples

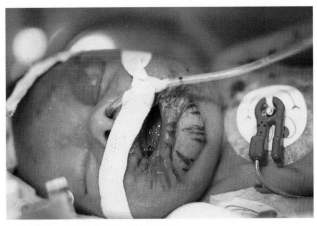

FIGURE 13–56. Pemphigus foliaceus

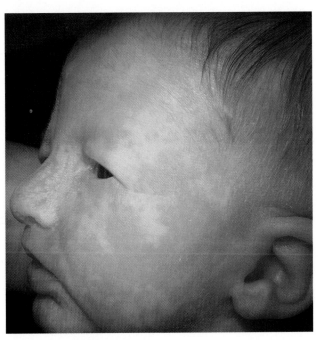

FIGURE 13–57. Goltz syndrome

SELECTED REFERENCES

Jones KL. (1997) Smith's Recognizable Patterns of Human Malformation. Philadelphia, WB Saunders.

Kuller JM and Lund CH. Assessment and management of integumentary dysfunction. *In* Kenner C, Brueggemeyer A, and Gunderson LP, Eds. (1993) Comprehensive Neonatal Nursing. Philadelphia, WB Saunders, pp 742–781.

Polin RA and Fox WW. (1998) Fetal and Neonatal Physiology. Philadelphia, WB Saunders, Chapters 71-77.

Solomon LM and Esterly NB. (1973) Neonatal Dermatology. Philadelphia, WB Saunders.

Taeusch HW and Ballard RA. (1998) Avery's Diseases of the Newborn. Philadelphia, WB Saunders, Chapters 105-109.

14 Neonatal Ophthalmology

The eye is the most complex sensory organ and the only organ in which most of the components can be examined. Table 14–1 details the development of the eye. The eye of a full-term baby is not completely developed functionally or anatomically.

The major ocular malformations (anophthalmia, microphthalmia, and fusion of the eyes with holoprosencephaly) are all associated with significant maldevelopment of the brain. Many other defects, such as coloboma, cataracts, and glaucoma, are associated with a variety of syndromes, transplacental infections, and metabolic disease. The lack of an iris is associated with glaucoma, cataracts, and a high incidence of Wilms tumor. If the child has a deletion of the short arm of chromosome 11, the association between aniridia and Wilms tumor is as high as 90%. The eye of the preterm infant is still undergoing rapid development. At approximately 34 weeks' gestation, there is complete clearing of the vessels of the lens capsule. Chromatic vision for the color red first can be detected at 34 weeks' gestation. However, the retina is not yet fully formed and will complete its development in the majority of babies near term gestation. Approximately 2 weeks after a full-term birth, the lacrimal gland is functional and tears are shed.

Retinopathy of prematurity remains a significant problem for extremely low birth weight babies under less than 750 grams. The primary risk factor remains an incompletely formed retina that fails to differentiate properly. Various cytokines, tissue growth factors, nutrients, and angiogenic factors in concert produce an abnormal vascular response. It may progress to permanent retinal damage owing to scarring and retinal detachment.

TABLE 14–1

DEVELOPMENT OF THE EYE	
24 days	Optic evagination
30 days	Optic cup
34 days	Lens invagination
38 days	Lens detached
	Pigmentation of retina
44 days	Lens fibers
	Migration of retinal cells
52 days	Corneal body
	Lens near final shape
8 wks	Eyelids
10 wks	Iris, ciliary body
	Eyelids fuse
12 wks	Retina layered
26 wks	Eyelids open
38 wks	Lacrimal duct canalized
5 mon postnatal	Iris pigmentation complete
	Binocular vision

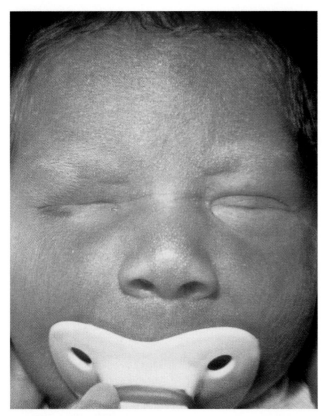

FIGURE 14–1. Anophthalmia

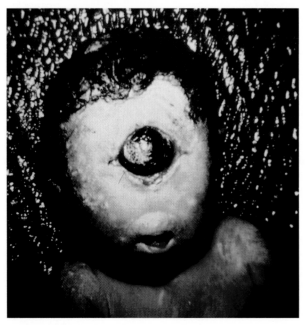

FIGURE 14–2. Cyclops—holoprosencephaly

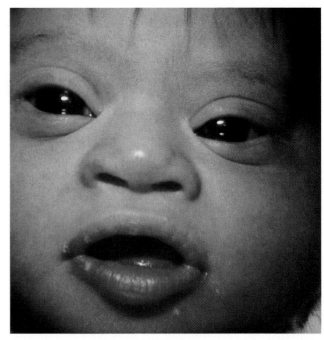

FIGURE 14–3. Wide-spaced eyes, epicanthal folds (trisomy 21)

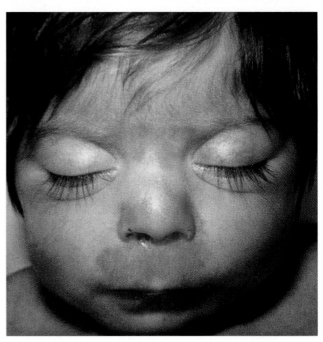

FIGURE 14–4. Long eyelashes—Cornelia de Lange syndrome

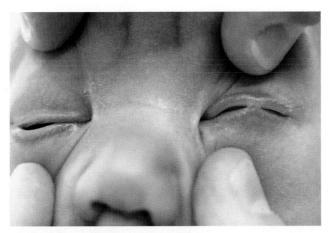

FIGURE 14–5. Partial fusion of eyelids

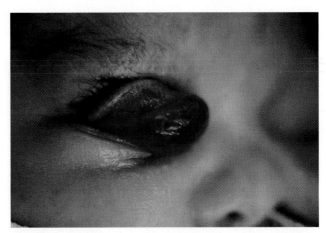

FIGURE 14–7. Hamartoma of the eyelid

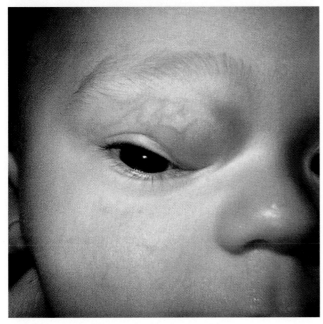

FIGURE 14–6. Eyelid hemangioma

EXSTROPHY OF GLOBES DUE TO MIDFACE BONY HYPOPLASIA

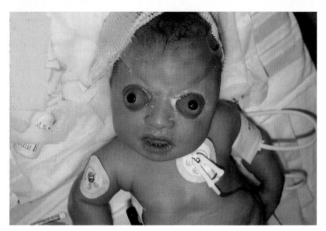

FIGURE 14–8. Frontal view

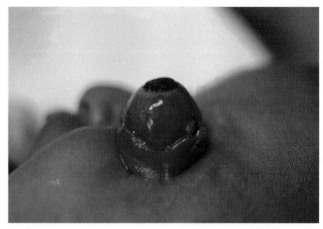

FIGURE 14–9. Lateral view with protruding globes

SCLERA

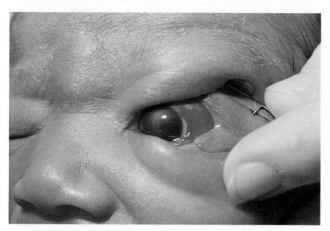

FIGURE 14–10. Traumatic scleral hemorrhage

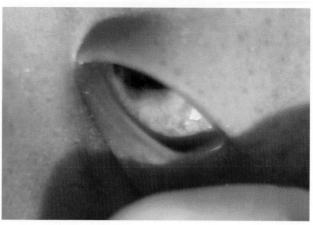

FIGURE 14–11. Scleral dermoid

ANTERIOR CHAMBER

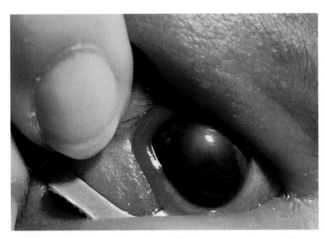

FIGURE 14–12. Traumatic rupture of Descemet membrane with resultant glaucoma

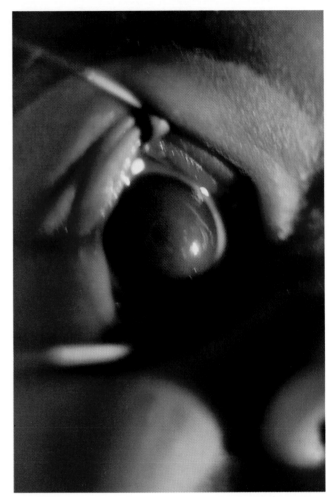

FIGURE 14–13. Primary glaucoma

IRIS

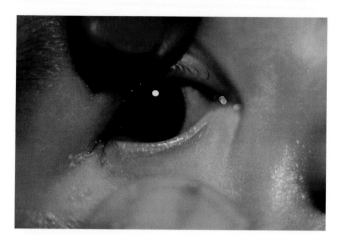

FIGURE 14–14. Aniridia

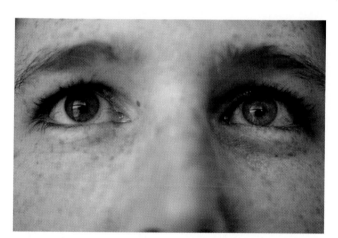

FIGURE 14–15. Heterochromia

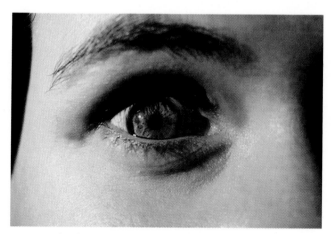

FIGURE 14–16. Heterochromia in a single iris—familial

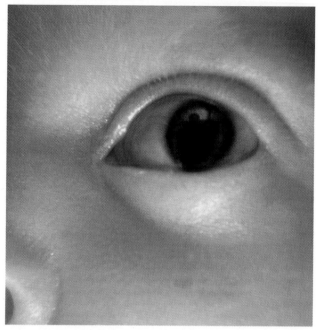

FIGURE 14–17. Coloboma

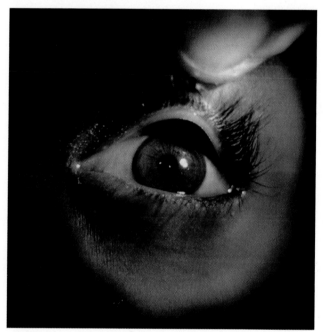

FIGURE 14–18. Kayser-Fleisher ring—Wilson disease

LENS—CATARACTS

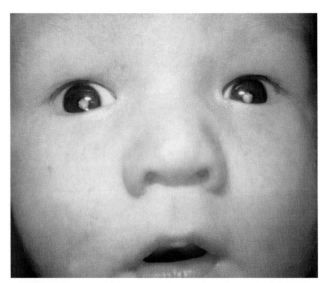

FIGURE 14–19. Central—familial

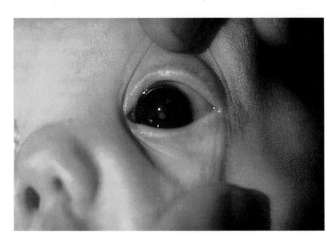

FIGURE 14–21. Smith-Lemli-Opitz syndrome

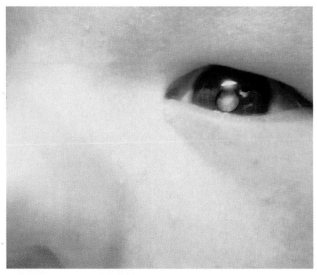

FIGURE 14–20. Cytomegalovirus

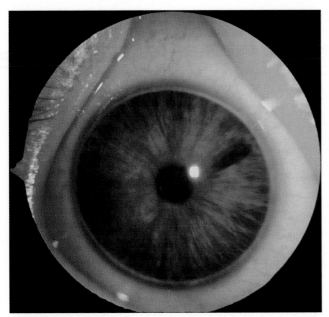

FIGURE 14–22. Axenfeld posterior embryotoxon

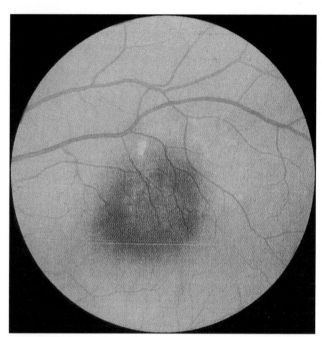

FIGURE 14–23. Benign choroidal nevus

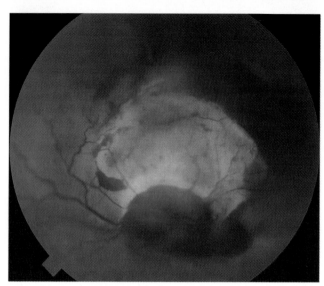

FIGURE 14–25. Hemorrhage with partial detachment

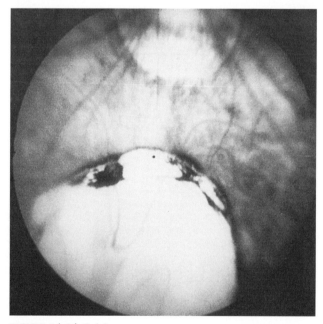

FIGURE 14–24. Coloboma

RETINOPATHY OF PREMATURITY

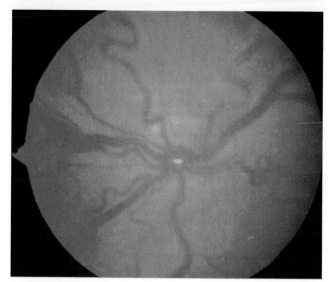

FIGURE 14–26. Vessel tortuosity

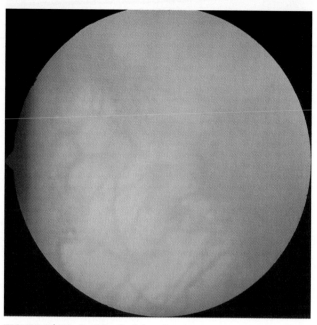

FIGURE 14–28. Partial retinal detachment

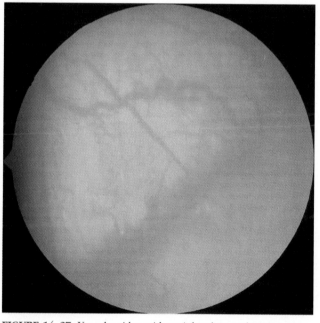

FIGURE 14–27. Vascular ridge with peripheral avascular zone

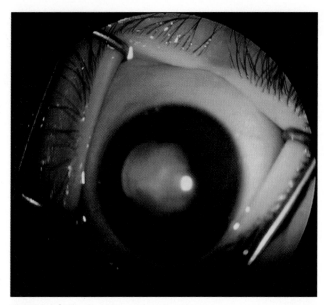

FIGURE 14–29. Complete retinal detachment

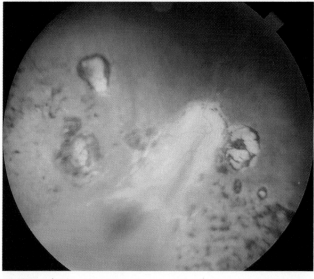

FIGURE 14–30. Old retinopathy—healed with scarring and evidence of traction on the vessels

OCULAR TUMORS

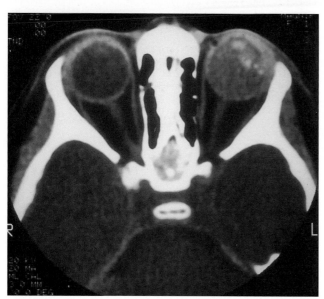

Retinoblastoma

FIGURE 14–31. Computerized tomography scan: intraocular calcifications

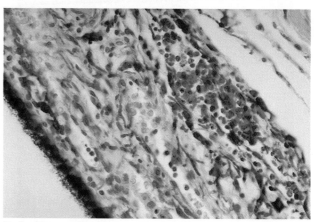

Retinoblastoma

FIGURE 14–33. Histology: numerous mitoses and rosettes of small, undifferentiated basophilic cells with little cytoplasm

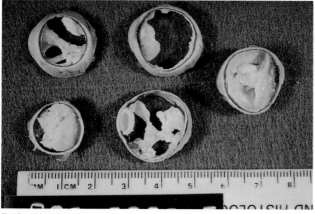

Retinoblastoma

FIGURE 14–32. Sections of globe

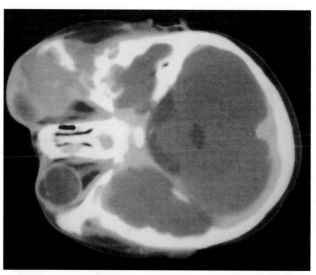

FIGURE 14–34. Rhabdomyosarcoma

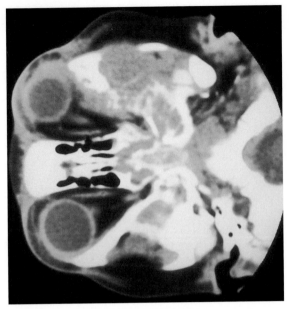

FIGURE 14–35. Metastatic neuroblastoma

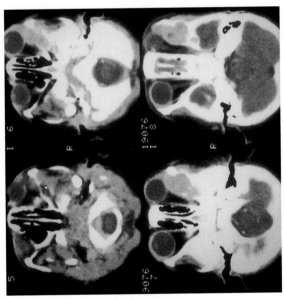

FIGURE 14–36. Hemangioendothelioma

SELECTED REFERENCES

Jones KL. (1997) Smith's Recognizable Patterns of Human Malformation, 5th ed. Philadelphia, WB Saunders.

Moore KL and Persaud TVN. (1993) The Developing Human, 5th ed. Philadelphia, WB Saunders.

Polin RA and Fox WW. (1998) Fetal and Neonatal Physiology, 2nd ed. Philadelphia, WB Saunders, Chapter 200.

Taeusch HW and Ballard RA. (1998) Avery's Diseases of the Newborn, 7th ed. Philadelphia, WB Saunders, Chapter 110.

Werner RB. Assessment and management of ophthalmic dysfunction. *In* Kenner C, Brueggemeyer A, and Gunderson LP, Eds. (1993) Comprehensive Neonatal Nursing. Philadelphia, WB Saunders.

15 Iatrogenic Problems

Iatros is the Greek word for a physician; therefore, iatrogenic refers to something that results from the activity of a physician. Originally the term was used in a much broader context, but it is now used in a limited manner to mean an adverse condition occurring as a result of treatment by a physician.

Newborn infants may be injured in many different ways. Initially, the process of birthing is forceful and traumatic. Molded heads and bruised faces and extremities are common events. Trauma may be inadvertently afflicted as part of appropriate patient care. The various electronic devices used to monitor and care for preterm infants all must be attached to the skin in some fashion. Cutaneous abrasions or blisters may develop at the site of attachment. In a similar fashion, some infants have a disproportionate reaction to agents used to cleanse the skin.

Some of the most dramatic injuries to neonates result from intravenous infiltrations or umbilical catheter accidents. These most commonly occur with less experienced nursing personnel who fail to recognize an intravenous (IV) infiltrate, thus allowing the IV fluid to accumulate in the tissue, promoting inflammation. Umbilical artery catheter accidents may occur from incorrect placement, but more commonly a medication is given inappropriately through the catheter, resulting in a severe ischemic process.

Insertion of endotracheal tubes or nasogastric tubes may result in trauma within the thorax. Since many of the complications relating to nasogastric tube placement or IV infiltrates do not involve physicians, the term iatrogenic is inappropriate. In that circumstance, the more appropriate term would be thalpogenic, which refers to the problem having been caused by a nurse (thalpos, Greek for an individual who cares for another).

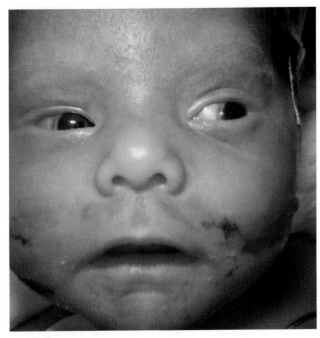

FIGURE 15–1. Facial abrasions from tape

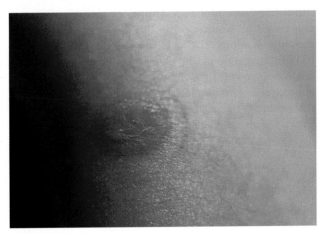

FIGURE 15–2. Suction catheter mark

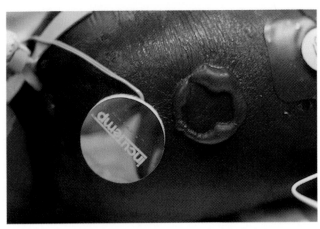

FIGURE 15–3. Electrode blister

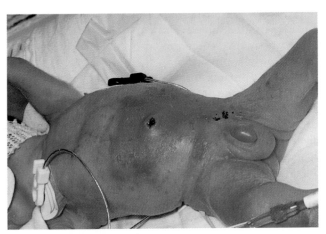

FIGURE 15–4. Povidone-iodine burn on abdomen

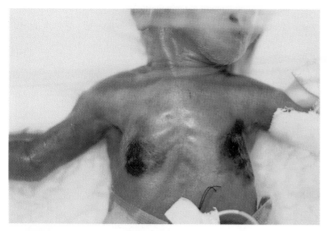

FIGURE 15–5. Electrode burns on chest

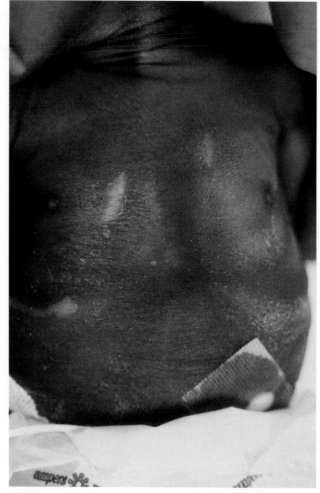

FIGURE 15–6. Chest abrasions, postinflammatory hypopigmentation

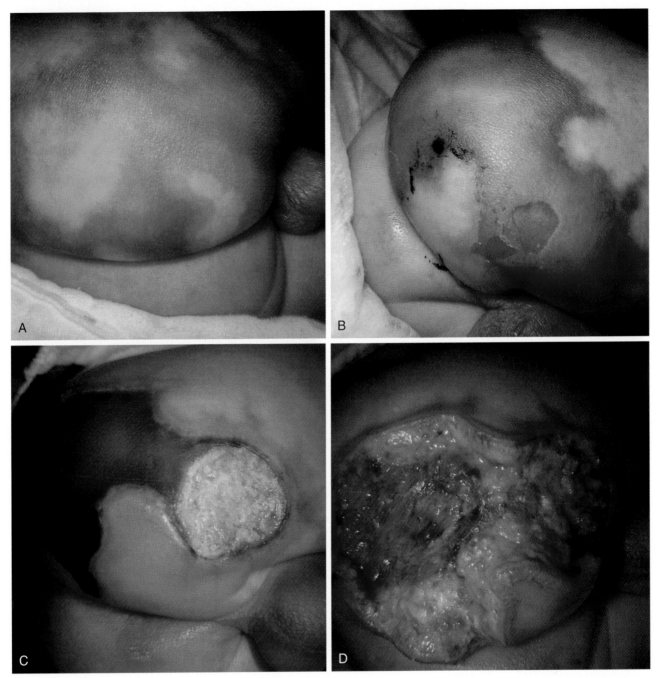

FIGURE 15–7. Umbilical artery catheter series: phenobarbital and benzodiazepine injected into an improperly located umbilical artery catheter. Initial ischemia proceeding to necrosis and scarring over 10 weeks: *A,* Day 1; *B,* Day 3; *C,* one week; *D,* 3 weeks.

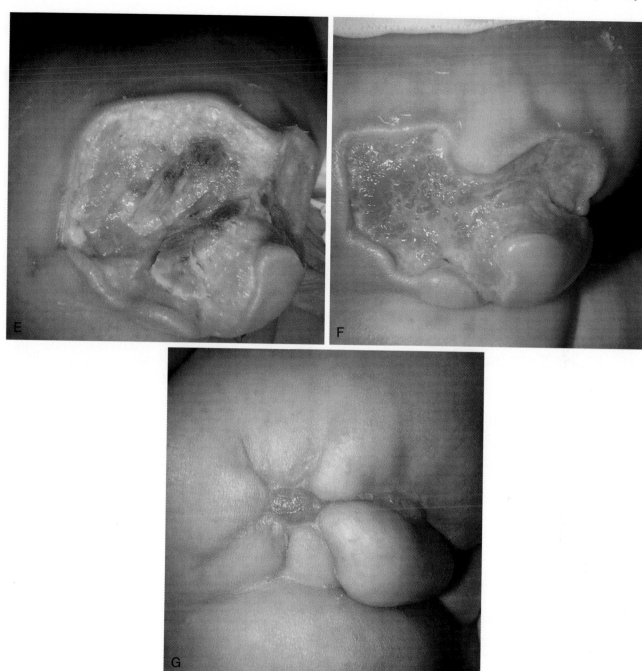

FIGURE 15–7, *continued. E,* 6 weeks; *F,* 8 weeks; *G,* 10 weeks.

INFILTRATES OF INTRAVENOUS SOLUTION

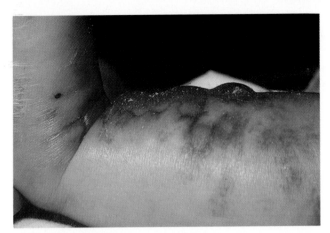

FIGURE 15–8. Parenteral solution infiltrate

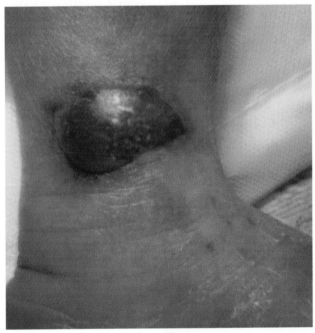

FIGURE 15–9. Calcium infiltrate, left ankle

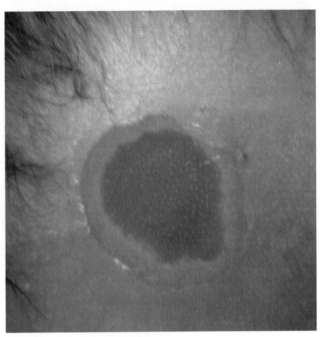

FIGURE 15–10. Medication infiltrate of scalp

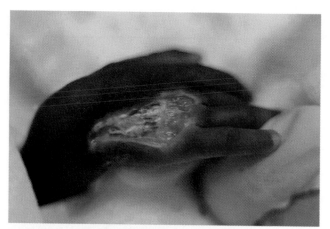

FIGURE 15–11. Deep tissue necrosis

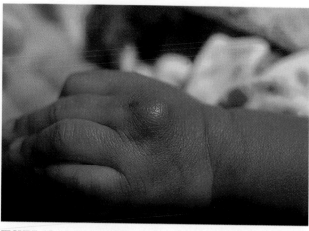

FIGURE 15–13. Inclusion cyst of the dorsum of the hand at the site of an old intravenous infiltrate

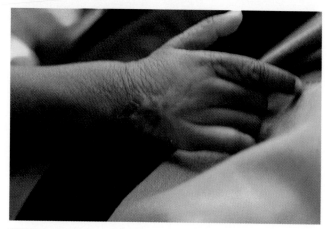

FIGURE 15–12. Scarred hand. Same child as in Figure 15-11.

ARTERIAL AND VENOUS CATHETERS

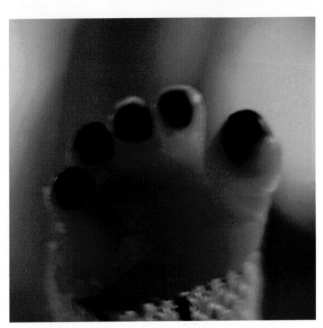

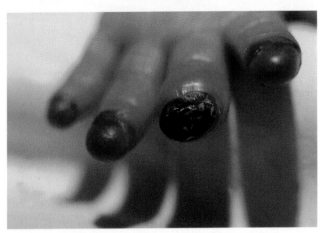

FIGURE 15–15. Necrosis of tips of the index finger and thumb from a radial artery catheter

FIGURE 15–14. Necrotic toes and fingers from umbilical artery catheter

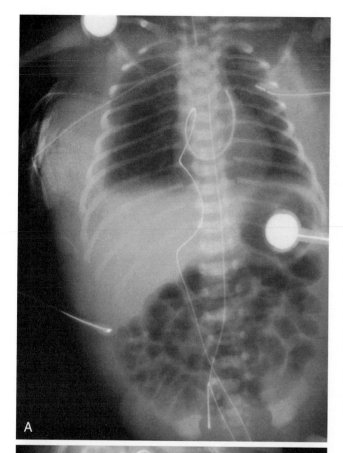

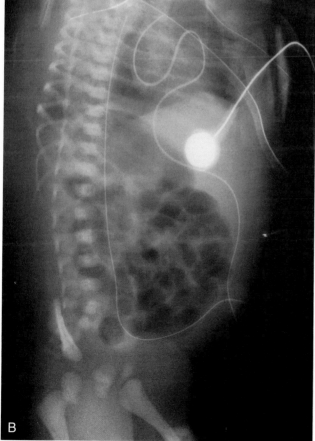

FIGURE 15–16. Umbilical venous catheter insertion into the pulmonary artery: (A) anteroposterior and (B) lateral views

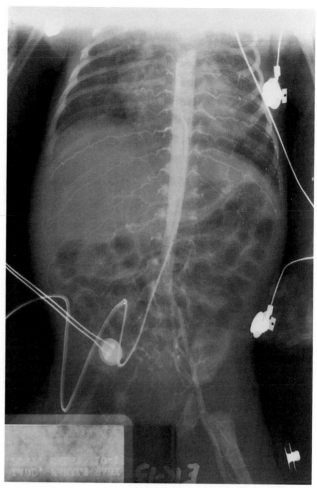

FIGURE 15–17. Aortic intima dissection from an umbilical artery catheter

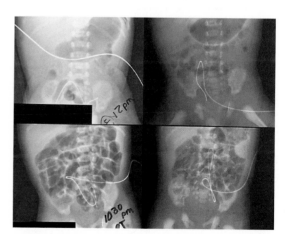

FIGURE 15–18. Four radiographs of improper placement of umbilical artery catheters

ESOPHAGEAL PERFORATION

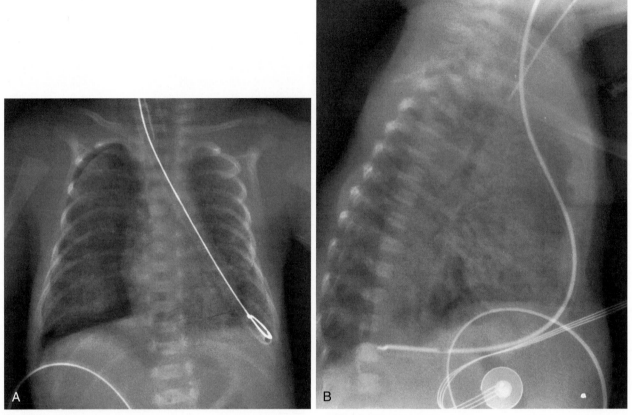

FIGURE 15–19. Esophagus perforated with nasogastric tube—catheter in the left hemithorax: (A) anteroposterior and (B) lateral views

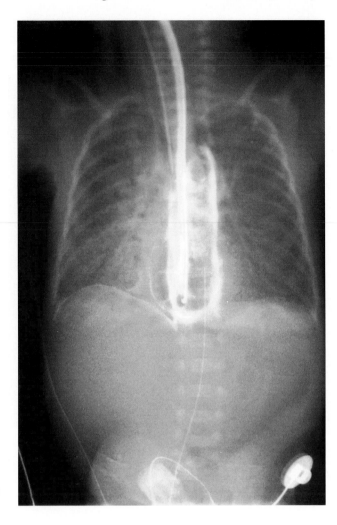

FIGURE 15–20. Esophageal perforation: paraesophageal extravasation of contrast material

LUNG INTUBATION—NASOGASTRIC TUBE

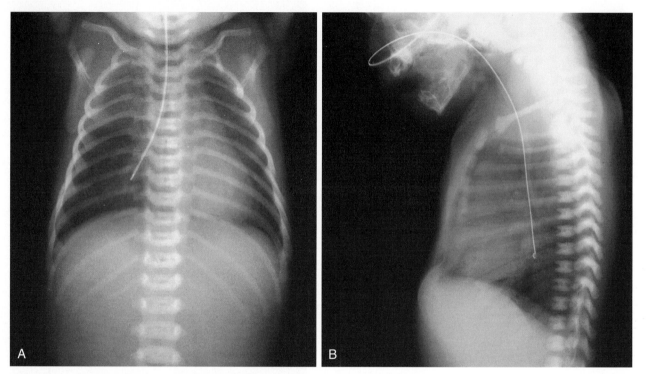

FIGURE 15–21. Nasogastric tube inserted into the right main stem bronchus with a right upper lobe infiltrate: (A) anteroposterior and (B) lateral views

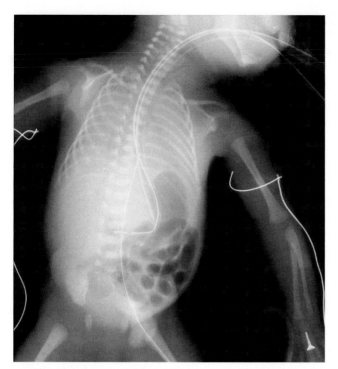

FIGURE 15–22. Gastric intubation

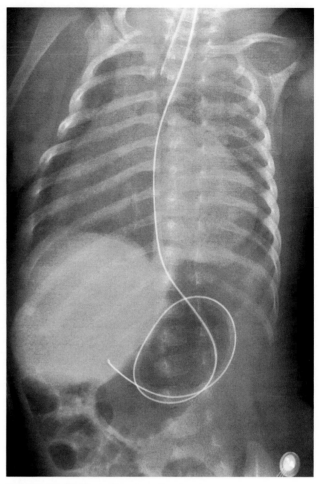

FIGURE 15–23. Knotted nasogastric tube

RIGHT PLEURAL EFFUSION

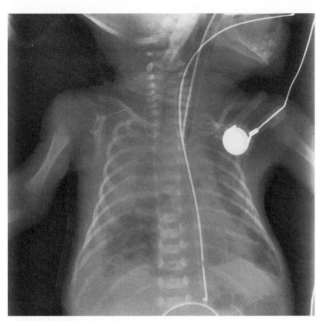

FIGURE 15–24. Accumulation of parenteral nutrition solution in the right hemithorax

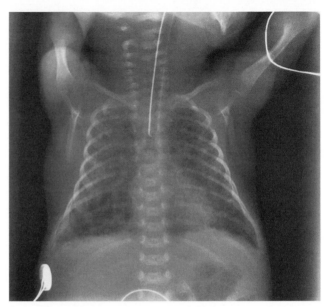

FIGURE 15–25. Resolution via thoracentesis

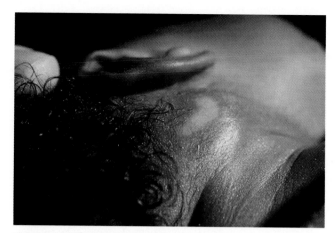

FIGURE 15–26. Subcutaneous fat necrosis of neck

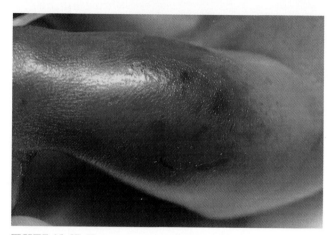

FIGURE 15–27. Hematoma at vitamin K injection site

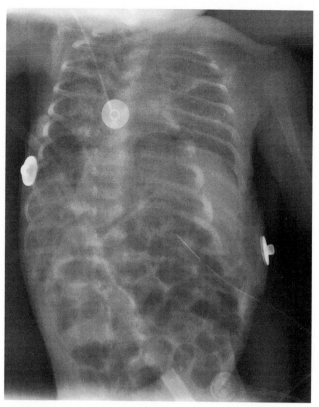

FIGURE 15–28. Radiographic double exposure of two babies

SELECTED REFERENCES

Jain L and Vidyasagar D. (1989) Iatrogenic Disorders in Modern Neonatology. Clin Perinatol 16:2.

Lefrak-Okikawa L. Iatrogenic complications of the neonatal intensive care unit. *In* Kenner C, Brueggemeyer A, and Gunderson LP, Eds. (1993) Comprehensive Neonatal Nursing. Philadelphia, WB Saunders.

Taeusch HW and Ballard RA. (1998) Avery's Diseases of the Newborn. Philadelphia, WB Saunders, Chapters 30, 31.

Index

Note: Page numbers followed by the letter t refer to tables.